A Textbook of Therapeutic Modalities in Psychiatric Nursing

A Textbook of Therapeutic Modalities in Psychiatric Nursing

For BSc and MSc Students (As per the Syllabus of Indian Nursing Council)

Manisha Gupta
RN RM BSc (N) MA (Sociology) MSc (N)
Associate Professor
People's College of Nursing and Research Centre
The People's University
Bhopal, Madhya Pradesh, India

JAYPEE BROTHERS MEDICAL PUBLISHERS
The Health Sciences Publisher
New Delhi | London

Jaypee Brothers Medical Publishers (P) Ltd

Headquarters
EMCA House
23/23-B, Ansari Road, Daryaganj
New Delhi 110 002, India
Landline: +91-11-23272143, +91-11-23272703
+91-11-23282021, +91-11-23245672
E-mail: jaypee@jaypeebrothers.com

Corporate Office
4838/24, Ansari Road, Daryaganj
New Delhi 110 002, India
Phone: +91-11-43574357
Fax: +91-11-4357 4314
E-mail: jaypee@jaypeebrothers.com

Overseas Office
J.P. Medical Ltd
83 Victoria Street, London
SW1H 0HW (UK)
Phone: +44 20 3170 8910
E-mail: info@jpmedpub.com

EU GPSR Authorised Representative
Logos Europe, 9 rue Nicolas Poussin
17000, La Rochelle, France
Phone: +33 (0) 6 67 93 73 78
E-mail: Contact@logoseurope.eu

Website: www.jaypeebrothers.com
Website: www.jaypeedigital.com

Inquiries for bulk sales may be solicited at: jaypee@jaypeebrothers.com

A Textbook of Therapeutic Modalities in Psychiatric Nursing

First Edition: 2015, *Reprint:* **2025**

ISBN 978-93-5152-354-3

Printed in India

Dedicated to

My husband and parents

Preface

Psychiatry is a very important branch of medicine. It is not only important for a nurse in training because it is a subject in nursing curriculum, but also because nursing students can apply these principles in any branch of medicine while dealing with patients. Psychiatric nursing is now evolving as a specialty in nursing. This book is written keeping the student nurse, a practicing nurse and a specialist nurse in mind. It is helpful for a student to pass her examination, the qualified nurse to practice her art better, and for a psychiatric nurse as a ready-reference book.

A Textbook of Therapeutic Modalities in Psychiatric Nursing is prepared according to the syllabus of Indian Nursing Council to enable the graduate and postgraduate students to use the therapies for various psychiatric disorders.

This book includes a unit on different therapies in psychiatric nursing for treating various psychiatric disorders. It covers introduction, definition, setting, types, purposes, advantages and disadvantages, and role of psychiatric nurse in various therapies and unit V also includes alternative therapies in psychiatry.

I have always loved teaching. I am glad to have been able to put down what I have always thought the nursing students ought to know about psychiatric therapies. My objectives will be fulfilled if this book helps the nurses to perform well in the clinical practices and examinations and caring for their patients.

Manisha Gupta

Acknowledgments

There are several hands and hearts behind this work. This final concrete shape of the book cannot be achieved without an optimal inspiration during this period, for which I would like to express my heartfelt gratitude.

On completion of the book with a sense of immense relief and satisfaction, I would like to express my heartfelt gratitude to all those who have assisted me and inspired me to achieve this goal.

Special acknowledgment should be made for the valuable assistance given by many people during the preparation of the book.

I would like to express my deep gratitude to Shri Jitendar P Vij (Group Chairman), Mr Ankit Vij (Group President) and Mr Tarun Duneja (Director–Publishing) of M/s Jaypee Brothers Medical Publishers (P) Ltd, New Delhi, India, for being instrumental in translating an idea mooted long ago into print, and also for providing nursing students with a book on therapies in psychiatric nursing in line with their syllabus.

I thank my husband, Mr Dilip Gupta, for the constant encouragement motivation and for doing computer work of typing which strengthened my resolve to come out with this publication.

I am also grateful to my friends and family members for the extensive help.

Last but not the least, I extend my thanks to all those who have directly or indirectly contributed in this work at various levels and whose names are not possible to be mentioned in the acknowledgments.

Contents

Introduction

Various causes may lead to varied mental illness. The treatment for specific illness differs from individual to individual. For the management of the client with psychiatric illness one or more methods will be used concurrently depending upon nature of illness, clinical manifestation and the behavior of the client.

- **Aims of Therapeutic Modalities**

1. To relieve the signs and symptoms
2. To promote recovery
3. To correct psychopathology
4. To rehabilitate the client in his own setting either in the community or in social group
5. To prevent relapse
6. To treat the patient as early as possible.

- **Classification of Therapeutic Modalities**

Unit–I. Psychopharmacotherapies

1. Antipsychotics
2. Antidepressants
3. Mood-stabilizing drugs
4. Anxiolytics (Antianxiety drugs)
5. Sedatives and hypnotics
6. Antiparkinsonism agents
7. Antabuse drugs
8. Drugs used in child psychiatry.

Unit–II. Psychological therapies

9. Individual psychotherapy
10. Group psychotherapy and supportive psychotherapy
11. Family therapy
12. Behavior therapy
13. Hypnosis or hypnotherapy
14. Narcoanalysis
15. Milieu therapy
16. Therapeutic community.

Unit–III. Somatic (physical) therapies

17. Electroconvulsive therapy
18. Psychosurgery.

UNIT-I
Psychopharmacotherapies

- Antipsychotics
- Antidepressants
- Mood-stabilizing Drugs
- Anxiolytics (Antianxiety Drugs)
- Sedatives and Hypnotics
- Antiparkinsonism Agents
- Antabuse Drugs
- Drugs used in Child Psychiatry

INTRODUCTION

Psychopharmacology is the study of drugs used to treat psychiatric disorders. It discusses many psycho-active medications that alter synaptic transmission in the brain in certain and specific ways. Medications that affect psychic function, behavior or experience are called psychotropic medications. They have significant effect on higher mental functions. Psychopharmacological agents are firstline treatment for almost all psychiatric ailments nowadays. Within the growing availability of a wide range of drugs to treat mental illness.

The invention of psychotherapeutic drugs has enacted a major change in the management of patient. The drugs are very effective in controlling the symptoms and return the patient to the community. Various drugs in psychiatry are called as psychotropic or psycho-active drugs.

HYSTORICAL PERSPECTIVES

Historically reaction to and treatment of the mentally ill ranged from begin involvement to intervention some would consider inhumane.

Individuals with mental illness were feared because of common beliefs associate them with demons or the supernatural.

Beginning in the late 18th century, a type of 'moral reform' in the treatment of persons with mental illness began to occur. This resulted in the establishment of community and state hospitals concerned with the needs of persons with mental illness. The early part of the 20th century scout the advent of the somatic therapies in psychiatry. Individuals with mental illness were treated with insulin shock therapy, wet sheet packs, ice baths, electroconvulsive therapy and psychosurgery prior to 1950, sedative and amphetamines were the only significant psychotropic medications available.

Since 1950s, the development of psychopharmacology has expanded to include widespread use of antipsychotic, antidepressant, and antianxiety medications.

CLASSIFICATION OF PSYCHOTROPIC DRUGS

1. Antipsychotics
2. Antidepressants
3. Mood-stabilizing drugs
4. Anxiolytics and hypnosedatives
5. Antiepileptic drugs
6. Antiparkinson drugs
7. Miscellaneous drugs which include stimulants, drugs used in eating disorders, drugs used in deaddiction, drugs used in child psychiatry, vitamins, calcium channel blockers, etc.

Chapter 1

Antipsychotics

INTRODUCTION

Antipsychotic agents are also known as neuroleptics, major tranquilizers or phenothiazines, this group of drugs has a major clinical use in the treatment of psychosis. Psychosis is a state in which a person's ability to recognize reality, to communicate and to relate to others is severely impaired (Wilson HA Kheisel).

The antipsychotic drugs are used to reduce the psychomotor excitement and control some symptoms of schizophrenia without causing disinhibition, confusion, sleep, hypnosis or anesthesia. The alternative terms of these drugs are neuroleptics, antischizophrenic, major tranquilizers.

The main therapeutic use of antipsychotic drug is to reduce hallucination, delusion, agitation, and psychomotor excitement in schizophrenia, organic psychosis and mania.

Antipsychotic drugs do not cure mental illness, but they calm the patient, relieve them, activate the immobile and withdrawn, and make some more accessible to psychotherapy.

Antipsychotics are those psychotropic drugs, which are used for the treatment of psychotic symptoms. These are also known as neuroleptics as they produce neurological side effects, major tranquilizers, D_2-receptor blockers and antischizophrenic drugs. This group of drugs are used to control the symptoms of psychosis. These drugs produce calming effect without significantly sedating the client.

For example: A typical antipsychotics = serotonin- dopamine antagonist. Namely as— Haloperidol (haldol), Chlorpromazine (Thorazine).

DEFINITION

Antipsychotic drugs are a class of medicines used to treat psychosis and other mental and emotional conditions.

HISTORY

The original antipsychotic drugs were happened upon largely by chance and were tested empirically for their effectiveness.

The first antipsychotic was chlorpromazine, which was developed as a surgical anesthetic, it was first used on psychiatric patients in the belief that it would have a calming effect. It was introduced for the treatment of psychosis during the period when lobotomy was a common treatment and was hailed as a 'cure' for schizophrenia. It was then touted to provide a 'chemical lobotomy', causing similar neurological effects without requiring surgery.

CLASSIFICATION

CLASSIFICATION OF ANTIPSYCHOTIC DRUGS

Class	*Drugs*	*Trade name*	*mg/day oral*	*IM(mg)*
Phenothiazines	Chlorpromazine	– Megatil – Largactil – Tranchlor	300 – 1500	50 – 100 IM only
	Triflupromazine	– Siquil	100 – 400	30 – 60 IM only
	Thioridazine	– Thioril, Melleril – Ridazin	300 – 800	
	Trifluoperazine	– Espazine	15– 16	1 – 5 IM 25 – 50 IM
	Fluphenazine	– Prolinate		every 1 – 3 weeks
Thioxanthenes	Flupenthixol	Fluanxol	3 – 40	
Butyrophen-ones	Haloperidol	– Senorm – Relinace – Serenace	5 – 100	5–20 IM
Diphenylbutyl	Pimozide	Orap	4 – 20	
Piperidines	Penfluridol	Flumap	20 – 60 Weekly	
Indolic derivatives	Molindone	Mobam	50 – 225	
Dibenzoxaze-pines	Loxapine	Loxapac	25 – 100	
Atypical anti-psychotic	– Clozapine	– Sizopin, Lozapin	50 – 400	
	– Risperidone	– Sizodon, Sizomax	2 – 10	
	– Olanzapine	– Oleanz	10 – 20 mg	
	– Quetiapine	– Qutan	150 – 750	
	– Ziprasidone	– Zisper	20 – 80 mg	
Others	Reserpine	Serpasil	0.5 – 50	

USAGE

Common conditions with which antipsychotics might be used include schizophrenia, mania and delusional disorder. They might be used to counter psychosis associated with a wide range of other diagnosis. Antipsychotics may also be used in mood disorder (e.g. bipolar disorder) even when no signs of psychosis are present.

INDICATIONS

1. **Organic Psychiatric Disorders**
- Delirium
- Dementia
- Delirium tremens
- Drug-induced psychosis and other organic mental disorders.

2. **Functional Disorders**
- Schizophrenia
- Schizoaffective disorders
- Paranoid disorders.

3. **Mood Disorders**
- Mania
- Major depression with psychotic symptoms.

4. **Childhood Disorders**
- Attention–deficit hyperactivity disorder
- Autism
- Enuresis
- Conduct disorder.

5. **Neurotic and Other Psychiatric Disorders**
- Anorexia nervosa
- Intractable obsessive—compulsive disorder
- Severe, intractable and disabling anxiety.

6. **Medical Disorders**
- Huntington's chorea
- Intractable hiccough
- Nausea and vomiting
- Tic disorder
- Eclampsia
- Heat stroke
- Severe pain in malignancy
- Tetanus.

PHARMACOKINETICS

The oral dose is absorbed erratically but with even blood level oral dose give peak level of 1½ hours, intramuscular administration gives more reliable blood level and peaks at 30 nots.

Since the antipsychotics are lipophilic, they easily enter into brain, kidneys, and lungs via blood. The dose is given based on the half-life drug.

The drugs are mainly metabolized in liver and excreted through kidneys. The effective/toxicity of the drug is based on the 'therapeutic window' of the drug.

- Antipsychotic when administered orally are absorbed variably from the gastrointestinal tract, with uneven blood levels.
- They are highly bound to plasma as well as tissue protein.
- Brain concentration is higher than plasma concentration.
- They are metabolized in liver, and excreted mainly through the kidneys. The elimination half-life varies from 10–24 hours.
- Most of the antipsychotic tend to have a therapeutic window. If the blood level is below this window, the drug is ineffective.

MECHANISM OF ACTION

- Antipsychotic drugs block D_2-receptors in the mesolimbic and mesofrontal systems (concerned with motioned reactions).
- Sedation is caused by alpha-adrenergic blockade.
- Antidopaminergic actions on basal ganglia are responsible for causing EPS (extrapyramidal symptoms).
- Atypical antipsychotics have antiserotonergic (5-hydroxyl-tryptamine or 5-HT). Antiadrenergic and antihistaminergic actions. These are therefore called as serotonin-dopamine antagonists.

MODE OF ACTION

The mechanism of action of antipsychotics is unknown. But, most probably, one of the major mechanism is the antidopaminergic activity of these drugs.

Antipsychotic drugs block D_2-receptors the dopamine receptors which are mainly present in the mesolimbic system (mesolimbic system is concerned with emotional reactions) and extrapyramidal system. The relative potencies of these drugs in competing for D_2-receptors parallel quite closely their clinical potencies.

The neurotransmitters (e.g. 5-HT, acetylcholine) are clearly implicated. The newer antipsychotics (called as SPA agents or serotonin dopamine antagonists) like risperidone, particularly act on the 5-HT_2 receptors.

Sedation is caused by histaminergic blockade, which is maximum for chlorpromazine and thioriodazine.

The antipsychotics, when administered to a psychotic patient, corrects this disordered thinking, difficulties in attention and concentration and perceptual abnormalities. In addition, the psychomotor activity becomes normal in both excited and withdrawn patients.

TYPICAL VS ATYPICAL COMPARISON

The atypical, second generation medications were marketed as offering greater efficacy in reducing psychotic symptoms while reducing side effects (and extrapyramidal symptoms in particular) than typical medications. These results showing these effects often lack robustness.

A study compared several atypical antipsychotics to an older typical antipsychotic perphenazine, among 1493 persons with schizophrenia. Perphenazine was chosen because of its lower potency and moderate side effect profile, the study found that only olanzapine outer performed perphenazine in the researchers principle outcome, the discontinuation rate. The apparent superior efficacy of olanzapine to the other drugs for greater reduction in psychopathology—Longer duration of successful treatment and lower rate of hospitalization for an exacerbation of schizophrenia. No other atypical studied (risperidone, quetiapine and ziprasodone) did better than the typical perphenazine on those measures. Olanzapine was associated with relatively severe metabolic effects; subject with olanzapine showed a major weight gain problem and increases in glucose, cholesterol and triglycerides, perphenazine did not create more extrapyramidal side effect, although more patients discontinued perphenazine owing to extrapyramidal effects compared to the atypical agents.

A subsequent phase was conducted dopamine indeed proved to be more effective at reducing medication drop-outs than other neuroleptic agents.

ATYPICAL ANTIPSYCHOTICS

1. **Clozapine (Clozaril)**—It requires weekly to biweekly CBC (FBC) because of risk of agranulocytosis (a severe decrease of white blood cells).
2. **Olanzapine (Zyprexa)**—It is used to treat psychotic including schizophrenia, acute manic episodes and maintenance of bipolar disorder. Dosing 2.5 mg–20 mg per day, comes in a form that quickly

dissolves in the mouth (Zyprexa zydis). It may cause appetite increase, weight gain and altered glucose metabolism leading to an increased risk of diabetes mellitus.

3. **Risperidone (Risperdal)**—Dosing 0.25 mg–6 mg per day and is titrated upward; divided dosing is recommended until initial titration is completed at which time the drug can be administered once daily. Available in long-acting form (Risperdal consta that is administered every 2 weeks; usual dose is 25 mg) comes in a form that quickly dissolves in the mouth (Risperdal of Tab) used off label to treat Tourette syndrome.
4. **Quetiapine (Seroquel)**—It is used primarily to treat bipolar disorder and schizophrenia, and 'off label' to treat chronic insomnia and restless legs syndrome; it is a powerful sedative (if it's used to treat sleep disorders and is not effective at 200 mg, it is not going to be effective in this regard).

   Dosing starts at 25 mg and continue upto 800 mg maximum per day, depending on the severity of the symptom(s)-being treated, users typically take smaller dose during the day for the neuroleptic properties and larger dose at bed time for the sedative effects, or divided in two equally high doses every 12 hours (75 mg – 400 mg bid).
5. **Ziprasidone (Geodon)**—Now (2006) approved to treat bipolar disorder. Dosing 20 mg twice daily initially upto 80 mg twice daily, prolonged QT interval a concern; watch closely with patients who have heart disease; when used with other drugs that prolong QT interval potentially life-threatening.
6. **Amisulpride (Solian)**—Selective dopamine antagonist, higher doses (greater than 400 mg) act upon postsynaptic dopamine receptors resulting in a reduction in the positive symptoms of schizophrenia, such as psychosis lower doses however act upon dopamine autoreceptors, resulting in increased dopamine transmission, improving the negative symptoms of schizophrenia.
7. **Paliperidone (Invega)**—Derivative of risperidone. Approved in December, 2006.

Dopamine partial agonists—

- i. Aripiprazole (Abilify)—Dosing 5 mg upto maximum of 30 mg has been used. Mechanism of action is thought to reduce susceptibility to metabolic.
- ii. Under clinical development—Bifeprunox, norclozapine.

CLASSIFICATION AND PROPERTIES OF ANTIPSYCHOTICS

TYPICAL ANTIPSYCHOTICS

Class and E.g. of Drugs	*E.g. of trade names*	*Oral dose range (mg/day)*	*Parental dose range (mg)*	*Equivalent dose (equal to sedation 100 mg of CPZ)*	*Common sedation*	*Side effects Hypotension*	*Eps (extrapyramidal symptoms)*
I. PHENOTHIAZINES							
A. Allpbatics							
1. Chlorpromazine (CPZ)	Megatil	300–2500	50–100 mg IM only	100	Severe	Severe	Mild
2. Triflupromazine	Siquil	100–400	30–60 IM	25	Moderate	Moderate	Moderate
B. Piperidines							
1. Thionidozine	Thioril	300–800	–	100	Severe	Moderate	Mild
C. Piperozines							
1. Triferoperozine	Espazine	15–60	1–5 IM	5	Mild	Mild	Severe
2. Prochlorperazine	Stemetil	45–150	40–80 IM	15	Mild	Mild	Severe
3. Fluphenazine hydrochloride	Anatensol	5–30	–	15	Mild	Mild	Severe
4. Fluphenazine decanoate	Prolinate	–	25–50 IM Every 13 weeks	6.7 (for 25 mg is given every 2 weeks)			
5. Thioproperazine	Majeptil	15–45	–	5	Mild	Mild	Severe

Contd...

Contd...

Class and E.g. of Drugs	*E.g. of trade names*	*Oral dose range (mg/day)*	*Parental dose range (mg)*	*Equivalent dose (equal to sedation 100 mg of CPZ)*	*Common sedation*	*Side effects Hypotension*	*Eps (extrapyramidal symptoms)*
II. THIOXANTHENES							
A. Aliphatics							
1. Chlorprothixene	(Taractan)	75–600	25–75 IM	50	Severe	Moderate	Moderate
B. Piperazines							
1. Thiothixene	(Navane)	6–60	2–6 IM	6	Mild	Moderate	Moderate
2. Flucothixol	Fluanxol	3–40	–	–	Probable	Probable	Mild
3. Flupenthixol decanoate	Fluanxol	–	20–40 IM every 2–4 weeks	40 mg every 2 weeks = 25 mg decanoate every 2 wks	Probable	Probable	Mild
III. BUTYROPHENONES							
1. Haloperidol	Senoem	5–100	5–20 IM	2	Mild	Mild	Severe
2. Haloperidol decanoate	Senoem LA	–	25–250 IM	100 mg every 4 weeks = 5 mg/day of Haloperidol	Mild	Mild	Severe
3. Trifluperidol	Triperidol	0.5–8.0 IM	2.5–5.0 IM	0.6	Probable	Probable	Severe

Contd...

Contd...

Class and E.g. of Drugs	*E.g. of trade names*	*Oral dose range (mg/day)*	*Parental dose range (mg)*	*Equivalent dose (equal to sedation 100 mg of CPZ)*	*Common sedation*	*Side effects Hypotension*	*Eps (extrapyramidal symptoms)*
IV. DIPHENYLBUTYL-PIPERIDINES							
1. Primozide	Oral	4–20	–	2	Mild	Mild	Moderate
2. Profluridol	Flumap	20–60 mg once every week	–	3.5 Probably for 20 mg given every week	Mild	Mild	Moderate
V. INOLIC DERIVATIVES (DIHYDROINDOLONES)							
1. Malindone	(Moban)	50–225	–	10	Moderate	0 (Obsces)	Mild
VI. DIBENZOXAZEPINES							
1. Loxapine	Loxapae	25–100	–	1	Mild	Mild	Moderate

SIDE EFFECTS OF ANTIPSYCHOTIC DRUGS

	Category	*Side effect*	*Action*	*Management*
1.	Autonomic side effects (ANS)	Dry mouth, constipation, cycloplegia, mydriasis, urinary retention, central anticholinergic syndrome tachycardia, orthostatic hypotension, impotence impaired ejaculation.	Blockade of muscarine cholinergic receptor	Usually tolerance develops. Otherwise treated with laxatives pilocarpine 2% diazepam, etc.
2.	Extrapyramidal side effects (EPS)	Parkinsonian syndrome (EPS tremor), akathisia (motor restlessness), acute dystonia, rabbit syndrome (perional tremor), tardive dyskinesia (oral facial), neuroleptic malignant syndrome.	Dopamine receptor Blockade	
3.	Central nervous system side effects	Seizure, sedative, depression, pseudodepression drowsiness, dizziness, lethargy, fatigue.	Adrenergic blockade, reduced catecholamine level	Decrease the dose, then continue
4.	Metabolic and endocrine side effect	Weight gain, galactorrhea, amenorrhea, increased appetite, glycosuria	Dopaminergic blockade leads to prolactine secretion	Change of drugs
5.	Allergic side effects	Cholestatic jaundice, agranulocytosis	Hypersensitivity	Stop the drug
6.	Cardiac side effects	EKG changes, sudden death	Anticholinergic effect	Change the drugs
7.	Ocular side effects	Granular deposit in cornea and in lens, pigmentary retinopathy, blurred vision.		Reduce the dose or change the drug
8.	Dermatological side effects	Contact dermatitis, photosensitive reaction, blue gray discoloration, pruritus, eczema, erythema		Reduce the dose or change the drug
9.	Miscellaneous	Fever, muscle stiffness, decreased sweating, nasal congestion, pale skin		Reduce the dose or change the drug

CONTRAINDICATIONS

Antipsychotics are contraindications in children under three years of age, comatose patients, patient with drug hypersensitivity, severe depression, and bone marrow depression.

NURSES RESPONSIBILITIES

1. Nurses should be aware of the side effects of the antipsychotic drugs and observe for the same in the patients.
2. If she observe early EPS symptoms, she should inform the doctor and injection phenergan may be given in severe form. For mild EPS tab. Pacitane 2 mg may be given.
3. Maintain vital chart.
4. For female, look for breast enlargement and maintain menstrual charting.
5. Weekly weight record should be maintained.
6. Watch for neuromalignant syndrome which is a serious problem.
7. When patients are on a typical antipsychotics watch for agranulocytosis.
8. Any infections should be recognized and taken care in time.
9. Advise the patient to get up slowly from squatting lying down position.

HALOPERIDOL

Haloperidol is a typical antipsychotic, it is in the butyrophenone class of antipsychotic medications and has pharmacological effects similar to the phenothiazines.

Haloperidol is a primitive antipsychotic used in the treatment of schizophrenia and more acutely, in the treatment of acute psychotic states and delirium. A long-acting decanoate ester is used as a long-acting injection given every 4 weeks to people with schizophrenia or related illness who have a poor compliance with medication and suffer frequent relapses of illness.

It was developed in 1957 by the Belgian company Janssen Pharmaceutica and submitted to first clinical trials in Belgium in the same year.

Pharmacology

Haloperidol is a neuroleptic and butyrophenone. Due to its strong control antidopaminergic action, it is classified as a highly potent neuroleptic. Haloperidol possesses a strong activity against delusions and hallucinations. Most likely due to an effective dopaminergic receptor blockage in the mesocortex and the limbic system of the brain. It blocks the dopaminergic action in the nigrostriatal pathways, which is the probable reason for the high frequency of extrapyramidal myotonic side effects (dystonia, akathisia, pseudoparkinsonism) it has minor antihistaminic and anticholinergic properties, therefore cardiovascular and anticholinergic side effects such as hypotension, dry mouth, constipation, etc. are seen quite infrequently, compared with less potent neuroleptics such as chlorpromazine. Haloperidol also has sedative properties and display a strong action against psychomotor agitation but due to a specific action in the limbic system it is therefore is an effective treatment for mania and states of agitation. Additionally it can be given as an adjuvant in the therapy of severe chronic pain.

The peripheral antidopaminergic effects of haloperidol account of its strong antiemetic activity. There it acts at the chemoreceptor trigger zone (CTZ). Haloperidol is useful to treat severe forms of nausea/emesis such as those resulting from chemotherapy.

Pharmacokinetics

Intramuscular injections

The drug is well and rapidly absorbed and has a high bioavailability plasma levels reach their maximum within 20 minutes after injection.

Intravenous injections

The bioavailability is 100% and the very rapid onset of action is seen within about ten minutes, the duration of action is 3–6 hours. If haloperidol is given as slow IV infusion, the onset of action is retarded, but the duration prolonged compared to 1 mg injection.

Therapeutic concentration

Plasma levels of 4 micrograms per liter to 20 (upto 25) micrograms per liter are required for therapeutic action. The determination of plasma levels can be used to calculate dose adjustments and to check compliance, particularly in long-term patients.

Uses

Haloperidol has found it to be an effective agent in treatment of symptoms associated with schizophrenia. Haloperidol is also used in the control of the symptoms of—

1. Acute psychosis, such as drug psychosis (LSD, amphetamines, ketamine and phencyclidine) psychosis associated with high fever or metabolic diseases.
2. Acute manic phases until the concomitantly given firstline drugs such as lithium or valproate are effective.
3. Hyperactivity, aggression.
4. Acute delirium.

5. Otherwise uncontrollable severe behavioral disorders in children and adolescents.
6. Agitation and confusion associated with cerebral sclerosis.
7. Adjunctive treatment of alcohol and opioid withdrawal.
8. Treatment of neurological disorders such as tic disorder, Tourette syndrome and chorea.
9. Treatment of severe nausea/emesis (postoperative, side effects of radiation and cancer chemotherapy).
10. Adjunctive treatment of severe chronic pain, always together with analgesics.
11. Therapeutic trial in personality disorders such as borderline personality disorders.
12. Also used in the treatment of intractable hiccups.

Contraindications

Absolute

- Pre-existing coma, acute stroke.
- Severe intoxication with alcohol or central depressant drugs.
- Known allergy against haloperidol or other butyrophenones or other drug ingredients.
- Known heart disease, when combined will tend towards cardiac arrest.

Special caution needed

- Pre-existing Parkinson's disease.
- Patients at special risk for the development of QT prolongation.
- Compromised liver function.
- Haloperidol may decrease the seizure—Threshold. Treat patients with epilepsy and those with risk factors for the development of seizures with caution. Maintain existing anticonvulsive therapy.
- Patients with hyperthyreosis; the action haloperidol is intensified and side effects are more likely, initiate an effective therapy of hyperthyreosis.
- IV injections: Inject slowly to avoid hypotension or orthostatic collapse. Avoid IV injections in cardiovascular unstable patients (preexisting hypotension, shock, concomitant antihypertensive therapy, heart insufficiency) prefer in these cases moderate oral or 1 mg doses.

Adverse Effects

The drug is noted for its strong early and late extrapyramidal side effects. The risk of the facial disfiguring tardive dyskinesia is around 4% per year in younger patients, higher than with most other antipsychotic drugs. Other predispositive factors may be female gender, pre-existing affective disorder and cerebral dysfunction.

Akathisia manifests itself with anxiety, dysphasia and an inability to remain motionless, other side effects include dry mouth lethargy, restlessness of akathisia, muscle-stiffness, muscle-cramping, restlessness, tremors and weight gain. Depression, severe enough to result in suicide is quite often seen during long-term treatment. Fatal neuroleptic malignant syndrome (NMD) is a significant possible side effect.

Pregnancy and Lactation

Unconfirmed studies is pregnant women revealed possible damage to the fetus, although most of the women were exposed to multiple drugs during pregnancy, following accepted general principles, haloperidol should only be given during pregnancy if the benefit to the mother clearly outweighs the potential fetal risk.

Haloperidol, when given to lactating women, is found to significant amounts in their milk. Breastfed children sometimes show extrapyramidal symptoms. If the use of haloperidol during lactation seems indicated, the benefit for the mother should clearly outweigh the risk for the child consider termination of breastfeeding.

Carcinogenicity

So far, no statistically acceptable evidence is found to associate long-term use of haloperidol with the potential for increased breast cancer risk in female patients.

Interactions

- Other central depressants (alcohol, tranquilizers, narcotics): Actions and side effects of these drugs.
- Methyldopa: Increased risk of extrapyramidal side effects and other unwanted central effects.
- Levodopa: Decreased action of levodopa.
- Tricyclic antidepressants: Metabolism and elimination of tricyclics significantly decreased, increased toxicity noted.
- Quinidine, buspirone and fluoxetine: Increased plasma levels of haloperidol, decrease haloperidol dose.
- Carbamazepine, phenobarbital and rifampicin.
- Lithium.
- Guanethiolene.
- Epinephrine.

Doses

As directed by the physician, depends on the condition to be treated, age and weight of patient.

Acute patients

Single doses of 1 mg – 5 mg (upto 10 mg) oral or, IM usually repeated every 4–8 hours. Do not exceed an oral dose of 100 mg daily. Doses used for IV injection are usually 5 mg – 10 mg as a single dose; not exceeding 50 mg daily.

Chronic conditions

0.5 mg – 20 mg daily oral, rarely more. The lowest dose that maintains remission should be employed.

Experimental doses

In resistant cases of psychosis small studies with oral doses of upto 300 mg – 500 mg daily have been conducted to avoid severe early extrapyramidal side effects.

Symptoms

Symptoms are usually due to exaggerated side effect. Most often encountered are—

1. Severe extrapyramidal side effects with muscle rigidity and tremors, akathisia, etc.
2. Hypotension or hypertension.
3. Sedation.
4. Anticholinergic side effects—Dry mouth, constipation, paralytic ileus, difficulties in urinating, massive sweating.
5. Coma in severe cases, accompained by respiratory depression and massive hypotension, shock.
6. Rarely serious ventricular arrhythmia.
7. Epileptic seizures.

Treatment

Treatment is merely symptomatic and involves intensive care with stabilization of vital functions. In early detected cases of oral overdose induction of emesis, gastric lavage and the use of activated charcol can all be tried. Avoid epinephrine for treatment of hypotension and shock because its action might be reversed.

Prognosis

Generally, the prognosis of overdose is good and lasting damage is not known, provided that the patient has survived the initial phase.

ADVERSE EFFECTS OF ANTIPSYCHOTIC DRUGS

I. Extrapyramidal symptoms (EPS):

These are the serious neurologic symptoms and major side effects of antipsychotic drugs.

- Neuroleptic-induced parkinsonism
  - Rigidity, tremors

- Bradykinesia
- Stooped posture
- Drooling
- Akinesia, ataxia.

- Acute dystonia
  - Involuntary movement
  - Opisthotonos
  - Oculogyric.
- Akathisia
  - Agitates
  - Restless and feel generally dysphonic.
- Tardive dyskinesia
  - Irregular choreoathetotic movements of the muscles of the head, limb and trunk.
- Neuroleptic malignant syndrome
  - Onset is often, but not invariably
  - Motor hypertonicity
  - Stiffness of the muscles in the throat and chest
  - The mental symptoms are akinetic mutism stupor.

II. Autonomic side effects:

- Dry mouth
- Constipation
- Cycloplegia
- Mydriasis
- Urinary retention
- Orthostatic hypotension
- Impotence and impaired ejaculation.

III. Seizures

IV. Sedation

V. Other effects

- Agranulocytosis (especially for clozapine)
- Sialorrhea or increased calivation (especially for clozapine)
- Weight gain
- Jaundice
- Dermatological effects (contact dermatitis, photosensitive reaction).

NURSE'S RESPONSIBILITY

- Instruct the patient to take sips of water frequently to relieve dryness of mouth.
- A high-fiber, increased fluid intake and laxatives if needed help to reduce constipation.
- Check BP before and after medication is given.
- Differentiate between akathisia and agitation and inform the physician.
- Observe the patient regularly for abnormal movements.
- Take all seizure precautions.

- Patient should be warned about driving a care operating machinery.
- Advise the patient to use sunscreen measures for photosensitive reaction.
- Teach the importance of drug complications, side effect, and regular follow-up.
- Seizure precaution should taught. Clozapine reduces seizure threshold.

Chapter 2

Antidepressants

INTRODUCTION

Antidepressants are those drugs which are used for the treatment of depressive illness. These are also called as mood elevators or thymoleptics. Antidepressants agents are used in affective disorders or disturbances mainly to treat depressive disorder caused by emotional and environmental stressors.

For example, tricyclic antidepressants (imipramine), tetracyclic antidepressants (maprotilene), monoamine oxidase inhibitors (isocarboxazid).

CLASSIFICATION

CLASSIFICATION OF ANTIDEPRESSANTS

Class	*Drugs*	*Trade name*	*Oral dosage mg/day*
Tricyclic antidepressants (TCAS)	– Imipramine	Antidep	75 – 300
	– Amitriptyline	Tryptomer	75 – 300
	– Clomipramine	Anafranil	75 – 300
	– Dothiepin	Prothiaden	
	– Mianserin	Depnon	30 – 120
Selective serotonin reuptake	– Fluoxetine	Fludac	10 – 80
Inhibitors (SSRIs)	– Sertraline	Serenata	50 – 200
Dopaminergic antidepressants	– Fluvoxamine	Faverin	50 – 300
Atypical antidepressant	– Amineptine	Servector	100 – 400
Monoamine oxidase	– Trazodone	Trazalon	150 – 600
Inhibitors[MAOIS]	– Isocarboxazid	Marplan	10 – 30

INDICATIONS

1. Depression
   - Depressive episode

- Dysthymia
- Reactive depression
- Secondary depression
- Abnormal grief reaction.

2. Childhood psychiatric disorders
   - Enuresis
   - Separation anxiety disorder
   - Somnambulism
   - School phobia
   - Night terrors.
3. Other psychiatric disorders
   - Panic attack
   - Generalized anxiety disorder
   - Agoraphobia and social phobia
   - OCD with or without depression
   - Eating disorder
   - Borderline personality disorder
   - Posttraumatic stress disorder
   - Depersonalization syndrome.
4. Medical disorders
   - Chronic pain
   - Migraine
   - Peptic ulcer disease.

Pharmacokinetics

- Antidepressants are highly lipophilic and protein bound.
- The half-life is long and usually more than 24 hours it is predominantly metabolized in the liver.

Mechanism of Action

The exact mechanism is unknown. The predominant action is by increasing catecholamine levels in the brain.

Side Effects

1. Autonomic side effects: Dry mouth, constipation, cycloplegia, mydriasis, urinary retention, orthostatic hypotension, impotence, impaired ejaculation, delirium.
2. CNS effects: Sedation, tremor and other extrapyramidal syndrome, seizures, jitteriness syndrome, precipitation of mania.
3. Cardiac side effects: Tachycardia, ECG changes, arrhythmias, direct myocardial depression.
4. Allergic side effects: Agranulocytosis, cholestatic jaundice, skin rashes.
5. Metabolic and endocrine side effects: Weight gain.

Nurse's Responsibility

- Patients on MAOIs should be warned against the danger of ingesting tyramine-rich foods which can result in hypertensive crisis. (beef liver, chicken liver, fermented sausages, dried fish, overripe fruits, chocolate and beverage like—Wine, beer and coffee).
- Report promptly if occipital headache, nausea, vomiting, chest pain or other unusual symptoms occur, these can herald the onset of hypertensive crisis.
- Restrict the patient not to take any medication without prescription.
- Strict monitoring of vitals, especially blood pressure is essential.

Chapter 3 Mood-stabilizing Drugs

INTRODUCTION

Bipolar disorder is a common recurrent and often severe psychiatric illness associated with high rates of morbidity and mortality if left untreated. Bipolar disorder also called manic-depressive disorder. Bipolar refers to the experience of both poles of mood: Mania and depression.

It is important to develop a comprehensive treatment plan for the patient with bipolar disorder including individual, family and psychosocial therapies is a critical component. The mood stabilizers include lithium. Valproate, carbamazepine, and other anticonvulsant mood stabilizers in the treatment of bipolar disorders.

Mood stabilizers are used for the treatment of bipolar affective disorders. Some commonly used mood stabilizers are:

- Lithium
- Carbamazepine
- Sodium valproate.

DEFINITION

Antimanic drugs are a class of medicines used to treat mania or manic phase of the bipolar disorders. It has also been used in the treatment of manic-depressive and schizoaffective disorders.

INDICATION

The major use of an antimanic agent is for treatment of mania and recurrent manic episodes.

DESIRED TREATMENT OUTCOMES

- Eliminate the symptoms of the mood episodes
- Stabilize the mood to prevent cycling between depression and mania
- Improve the client's self-care ability, function and quality of life.

MODE OF ACTION

The specific biochemical mechanism of action of antimanic agents is unclear.

Antimanic agents produce many neurochemical changes in the area of brain. These changes may affect norepinephrine and serotonin in the part of CNS involved in emotion. It may decrease the activity of the nerve impulse, resulting in depression or increase in the nerve impulse, causing mania.

Lithium also helps in maintaining the sodium concentration in the brain, thereby regulating the mood servings as well as impulse along the nerve cells.

CLINICAL AND PHARMACOKINETIC PARAMETERS OF MOOD STABILIZERS (ANTIMANIC AGENTS)

Generic name	*Brand name*	*Dosage range (mg/day)*	*Half-life (hrs).*	*Onset (days)*	*Duration*
Lithium	Eskalith Lithobid	Acute 1800 maintenance 400 – 1300	21 – 30	5 – 14 days	2 weeks
Toperamate	Topamax	Maintenance 400 – 1300	21		
Lamotrifine	Lamictal	Maintenance 300 – 500	29		
Valproic acid	Depakine	1200 – 2500	5 – 20		
Devalproex sodium	Depakote	1200 – 2500	5 – 20		

TARGET SYMPTOMS FOR MOOD-STABILIZING DRUG THERAPY

Mania, irritability, euphoria, expansiveness, manipulativeness, lability with depression, sleep disturbance (decreased sleep), pressured speech, flight of ideas, motor hyperactivity, assualtiveness/threatening behavior, distractibility, hypergraphia, hypersexuality, persecutory and religious delusions, geandiosity hallucinations, ideas of reference, catatonia.

ANTIMANIC DRUGS

Lithium

Lithium is a naturally occurring alkali metal that shows some characteristic with other monovalent cations such as sodium and potassium. In 1949, cade in Australia, was the first to report the therapeutic effects of lithium to treat mania.

Lithium is used to treat acute hypomanic or manic episodes and recurrent affective disorders. 70%–90% of client with typical bipolar illness respond to lithium.

Some times, lithium is used to treat schizoaffective disorders, often in conjunction with an antipsychotic agent. Lithium is been found to be effective in the treatment of aggressive or impulsive behaviors.

Lithium is an element with atomic number 3 and atomic weight 7. It was discovered by Fj Code in 1949, and is a most effective and commonly used drug in the treatment of mania.

Indications

Lithium salt used in treatment of a myriad of psychiatric and nonpsychiatric disorders—

1. R_x of acute mania
2. Prophylaxis of bipolar mood disorder
3. R_x of schizoaffective disorder
4. R_x of cyclothymia
5. R_x of acute depression
6. Chronic alcoholism
7. R_x of impulsive aggression
8. R_x of Kleine-Levin syndrome.

Other disorders are:

- Premenstrual dysphonic disorder
- Bulimia nervosa
- Borderline personality disorder.

Clinical use

Lithium is available in market in the form of the following preparations—

1. Lithium carbonate 300 mg tab. 400 mg sustained release tablet.
2. Lithium citrate 300 mg/5 ml liquid.

Before starting treatment, it is essential to make sure of normal functioning of kidneys thyroid, heart and CNS. After starting lithium it is necessary to investigate these systems at repeated intervals. Usual profile of investigation as follows:

1. Routine general and systemic physical examination
2. Routine blood counts (Hb, TC, DC, ESR)
3. Urine-routine and microscopic examination
4. EKG
5. Renal function tests (blood urea, serum creatinine, 24 hours urine volume, urine specific gravity). GFR with creatinine clearance test
6. Thyroid function test.

Pharmacokinetics

Lithium is readily absorbed with peak plasma levels occurring 2 – 4 hours after a single oral dose of lithium carbonate. Lithium is distributed rapidly in liver and kidney and more slowly in muscle, brain and bone. Steady-state levels are achieved in about 7 days. Elimination is predominantly via kidneys. Lithium is reabsorbed in the proximal tubules and is influenced by sodium balance. Depletion of sodium can precipitate lithium toxicity.

Mechanism of action

The probable mechanisms of action can be—

- Accelerates presynaptic re-uptake and destruction of catecholamines, like norepinephrine.
- Inhibits the release of catecholamines at the synapse
- Decreases postsynaptic serotonin receptor sensitivity.

The following mechanisms of action of lithium have been hypothesized.

1. If affects the Na^+– K^+– ATPase and accumulates intracellularly as a substitute of Na^+.
2. It inhibits the adenylate cyclase and thus decreases CAMP messenger intracellularly.
3. It accelerates the presynaptic reuptake and destruction, of catecholamines like norepinephrine.
4. It inhibits the release of catecholamines at the synapse.
5. It decreases the postsynaptic serotonin $5HT_2$ receptor sensitivity.
6. It stabilizes the cell membrane, along with Ca^{++} and Mg^{++}.
7. Decreases the Ca^{++} mobilization from the intracellular pools by inositol triphosphate dependent Ca^{++} channels.
8. It interferes with the phosphatidy-inositol cycle by blocking the conversion of inositol monophosphate to inositol by inositol monoposphate phosphatase. The muscarinic acetylcholine (ACh) receptor is among one of the neurotransmitter receptors linked to this system in brain. The antimanic effects of lithium may be attributed to this effect on ACh, thus affecting cholinergic-adrenergic balance.

   All these actions result in decreasing catecholamine activity, thus ameliorating mania.

Dosage

Lithium is available in the market in the form of the following preparations:

Lithium carbonate—300 mg tablets (lithcab), 400mg (lithoSUNSR)
Lithium citrate—300 mg/ 5 ml liquid.

Blood lithium levels

Therapeutic levels = 0.8–1.2 mEq/l (treatment for acute mania)
Prophylactic levels = 0.6–1.2 mEq/l (prevention of relapse in bipolar disorder)

Toxic lithium levels >2.0mEq/l.

Side effects

1. Neurological: Tremors, motor hyperactivity, muscular weakness, seizures, and neurotoxicity (delirium, abnormal involuntary movement).
2. Renal: Polydipsia, polyuria, tubular enlargement, and nephrotic syndrome.
3. Cardiovascular : T-wave depression.
4. Gastrointestinal: Nausea, vomiting, diarrhea, abdominal pain, and metallic taste.

5. Endocrine: Abnormal thyroid function, goiter, and weight gain.
6. Dermatological: Acneiform eruptions, popular eruptions, and exacerbation of psoriasis.
7. Lithium toxicity: Toxicity occurs when serum lithium level > 2.0 mEq /l.
8. Side effects during pregnancy and lactation:
   i. Teratogenic
   ii. Increased incidence of Ebstein's anomaly
   iii. Secreted in milk with 30% – 100% of maternal blood lithium levels can cause toxicity in infant.

Signs and symptoms of lithium toxicity

- Ataxia
- Coarse tremor (hand)
- Nausea and vomiting
- Impaired memory
- Impaired concentration
- Nephrotoxicity
- Muscle weakness
- Convulsions
- Muscle twitching
- Dysarthria
- Lethargy
- Confusion
- Coma
- Hyper-reflexia
- Nystagmus.

ADVERSE EFFECTS ASSOCIATED WITH LITHIUM THERAPY

Plasma level (mEq/l)	*Common side effects*	*Less common side effects*
<1.5	Initial R_x: fine hand tremors, polyurea, mild thirst, transcent and mild nausea and discomfort Afterwards: fatigue, acne, ECG changes, hypothyroidism	Twitching, muscular weakness restlessness dry mouth and thinning hair
1.5 – 2.0	Diarrhea, vomiting, nausea drowsiness, muscle weakness, lack of coordination	
2.0 – 3.0	Giddiness, ataxia, blurred vision, tinnitus, vertigo, increased confusion, slurred speech blackout, incontinence fasciculation, myoclonic	
> 3.0	Seizures, arrhythmias, hypotension, peripheral vascular collapse, stupor, spasticity	

Contraindications of lithium use

- Cardiac, renal, thyroid or neurological dysfunction
- Presence of blood dyscrasias
- During first trimester of pregnancy and lactation
- Severe dehydration
- Hypothyroidism
- History of seizures
- Presence of clear evidence of cardiac, renal thyroid or neurological dysfunction
- Presence of blood dyscrasia
- During first trimester of pregnancy and lactation
- Concomitant administration of thiazide, diuretics, tetracyclines or anesthetics.

Management of lithium toxicity

- Discontinue the drug immediately.
- For significant short-term ingestions, residual gastric content should be removed by induction of emesis, gastric lavage, and absorbtion with activated charcoal.
- If possible instruct the patient to ingest fluids.
- Assess serum lithium levels, serum electrolytes, renal functions, and ECG as soon as possible.
- Maintenance of fluid and electrolyte balance.
- In a patient with serious manifestations of lithium toxicity, and hemodialysis should be initiated.

Nurse's responsibilities

The prelithium work-up

A complete physical history, ECG, blood studies (TC, DC, FBS, BUN, creatinine, electrolyte), and urine examination (routine/micro) must be carried out. It is important to assess renal function as renal side effects are common and the drug can be dangerous in an individual with compromised kidney function.

To achieve therapeutic effect and prevent lithium toxicity, the following precautions should be taken

- Lithium must be taken on a regular basis, preferably at the same time daily (a patient taking lithium on TID schedule, who forgets a dose should wait until the next scheduled time to take lithium and not take twice the amount at one time as it can lead to lithium toxicity).
- When lithium therapy is initiates mild side effects such as find hand tremors, increased thirst and urination, nausea, and anorexia, may develop.
- Serious side effects of lithium that necessitate its discontinuance.
- Since polyuria can lead to dehydration with the risk of lithium intoxication, patient should be advised to drink enough water to compensate for the fluid loss.

- Frequent serum lithium level evaluation is important.
- Blood for determination of lithium level should be drawn in the morning approximately 12–14 hours after the last dose was taken.
- The patient should be told about the importance of regular follow-up.

Carbamazepine

Carbamazepine is an antimanic and mood-stabilizing agent. It is a tricyclic compound synthesized in 1953 by Schindler.

The onset of action is faster as compared to lithium, but slower compared to valproate 600 mg – 1600 mg/day orally is divided dose R_x is best monitored with repeated blood levels. The therapeutic blood levels are 6 mg – 12 mg/ml. The toxic blood levels are reached at more than 15 mg/ml.

It is available in the market under different tradenames like tegretol, mazetol, zeptol and zen retard.

Indications

- Seizures— Complex partial seizures, GTCS, seizures due to alcohol withdrawal.
- Psychiatric disorders— Rapid cycling bipolar disorder, acute depression, aggression, psychosis with epilepsy, schizo-affective disorders, personality disorder, cocaine withdrawal syndrome.
- Paroxysmal pain syndromes— Trigeminal neuralgia and phantom limb pain.

Dosage

The average daily dose is 600 mg – 1800 mg orally, in divided doses.
The therapeutic blood levels are 6 mg – 12 mg/ml. Toxic blood levels are attained at more than 15 mg/ml.

Mechanism of action

It is structurally related to imipramine. It enhances GABA activity in the brain and inhibits glutamate and aspartate activity. It possesses psychotropic effects and is less sedating thorn most anticonvulsants. The drug elevate mood in some depressed client and is a second line R_x for bipolar disorder.

Its mood-stabilizing mechanism is not clearly established. It anticonvulsant action may however be by decreasing synaptic transmission in the CNS.

Side effects

Major: Diplopia, drowsiness, dizziness, nausea, vomiting, ataxia, skin rash, photosensitivity, cholestatic jaundice, acute oliguria with hypertension, leukopenia, and thrombocytopenic purpura.

Most dangerous side effects: Bone marrow depression Cardiovascular collapse.

It is essential to monitor cardiac, renal, hepatic, and bone marrow functions during treatment.

Avoid during pregnancy and lactation.

- Drowsiness
- Ataxia
- Confusion
- Hypertension
- Headache
- Arrhythmias
- Skin rashes
- Nausea and vomiting, diarrhea
- Dry mouth
- Abdominal pain
- Oliguria
- Jaundice
- Leukopenia
- Hepatitis
- Thrombocytopenia.

Nurse's responsibilities

- Since the drug may cause dizziness and drowsiness advise him to avoid driving and other activities requiring alertness.
- Advise patient not to consume alcohol when he is on the drug.
- Emphasize the importance of regular follow-up visits and periodic examination of blood count and monitoring of cardiac, renal, hepatic and bone marrow functions.

SODIUM VALPROATE, ENCORATE, CHRONO, VALPARIN, EPILEX, EPIVAL

Oxcarbazepine

Effective as carbamazepine in the treatment of bipolar disorder. It should be considered an alternative for clients unable to tolerate carbamazepine.

Mechanism of action

Oxcarbazepine is the 10-keto, 11-dihydro-co-ox-carbazepine analog of carbamazepine.

Side effects

- Headache, drowsiness, dizziness, and ataxia

- Tremor, abnormal gait, fatigue, and sedation encephalopathy
- Hyperlipidemia, antidiuretic hormone effective allied reproductive hormones.

Lamotrifine

Used in bipolar depression and in rapid cycling bipolar disorders.

Lamotrifine requires a slow titration; the titration schedule must be followed to minimize risk of skin rash.

Side effects

- Headache
- Dizziness
- GI distress
- Blurred or double vision.

Dry interaction

- Interactions with valproate.

Gabapentin

Gabapentin (Neurontin) is a GABA analog. Gabapentin has been used for adjunctive therapy as a mood stabilizer and for the treatment of partial seizure in social phobia.

Gabapentin has many other uses including adjunctive therapy in alcohol detoxification, anxiety disorder, dystonia, essential tremor OC behavior, phantom limb syndrome, and pain management.

Absorption, distribution, metabolism and execution

The bioavailability of gabapentin decreased with increasing dose. Its bioavailability is approx 60% when dosed at 400 mg every 8 hours.

Bioavailability is reduced to 35% at a does of 1200 mg every 8 hours.

Less than 35% of gabapentin is protein bound drug is not metabolized but executed unchanged in wine.

Side effects

- Leukopenia
- Hypertension, vasodilation, edema, peripheral edema, and facial edema
- Fluctuations in blood sugar levels
- Ataxia, dizziness, involuntary movements, somnolence, and pruritic rash.

Topiramate

Topiramate is a sulfamate substituted monosaccharide and indicated for treatment of epilepsy.

Topiramate is also used in the treatment of binge eating, bulimia, cluster headache, and trigeminal neuralgia.

Absorption, distribution, metabolism and execution

- It is well-absorbed after oral doses peak serum concentration occur in 2–4 hours
- Food alters the rate of absorption
- Topiramate is minimally bound to protein
- Druff is not metabolized and is executed unchanged in urine.

Dosage

It should be treated slowly, initial dose of 50 mg/day, for 1st week and increased in 50 mg increments per week until a dose of 400 mg/day is reached.

Side effects

- Anemia
- Hypertension, postural hypotension, vasodilation arrhythmias, and palpitations
- Drowsiness, dizziness, ataxia, speech disorders, confusion, language problems, and anxiety
- Auditory hallucination.

Nurse's responsibility when patients are on antimanic drugs

1. Before lithium therapy. Excessive weight gain or swelling of ankles and wrists should be noted weekly weight record should be maintained.
2. Regular serum lithium level LFT (liver function test) and R_x (thyroid function test) to be monitored.
3. Monitor Na intake.
4. Above 40 years ECG to be done regularly.
5. Stop the drug if fluid loss occurs and then restart.
6. Activities which increases perspiration.
7. Careful monitoring of blood count to be done and any kind of infection to be notified early.
8. Advice the patient not to increase or decrease medicine unless advised.

Chapter 4

Anxiolytics (Antianxiety Drugs)

BENZODIAZEPINES

These are also called as minor tranquilizers. Most of them belong to the benzodiazepine group of drugs.

1. Barbiturates:
- Phenobarbital
- Pentobarbital
- Secobarbital
- Thiopentone.
2. Nonbarbiturate, nonbenzodiazepine, and antianxiety agents:
- Meprobamate
- Glutethimide
- Diphenhydramine
- Methaqualon.
3. Benzodiazepines: Presently benzodiazepines are the drugs of first choice in the treatment of anxiety, and for the treatment of insomnia.
- Very short-acting : Triazolam
  Midazolam
- Short-acting – Oxazepam (Serepax)
  – Lorazepam (Ativan, Trapex, Larpose)
  – Alprazolam(Restyl, Trika, Alzolam, Quiet)
- Long-acting – Chlordiazepoxide (Librium)
  – Diazepam (Valium, calmpose)
  – Clonazepam (Lonazep)
  – Flurazepam (Nindral)
  – Nitrazepam (Dormin).

Indications for Benzodiazepines

- Anxiety disorders
- Insomnia
- Depression
- Panic disorder and social phobia
- Obsessive compulsive disorder
- Posttraumatic stress disorder
- Bipolar-I disorder

- Other psychiatric indications include alcohol withdrawal, substance-induced and psychotic agitation.

Dosage (mg/ day)

- Alprazolam 0.5 – 6 mg/day PO
- Oxazepam 15 – 120 PO
- Lorazepam 2 – 6 PO/IV/IM
- Diazepam 2 – 10 PO /IM/ slow IV
- Clonazepam 0.5 – 20 PO/IM
- Chlordiazepoxide 15 – 100 PO, 50 – 100 slow IV
- Nitrazepam 5 – 20 PO.

Mechanism of Action

Benzodiazepines bind to specific sites on the GABA receptors and increase GABA level. Since GABA is an inhibitory neurotransmitter, it has a calming effects on the central nervous system, thus reducing anxiety.

Side Effects

- Nausea, vomiting, and weakness
- Vertigo, and blurring of vision
- Bodyaches, epigastric pain, and diarrhea
- Impotence, and sedation
- Increased reaction time
- Ataxia, dry mouth, and retrograde amnesia
- Impairment of driving skills
- Dependence and withdrawal symptoms.

Nurse's Responsibility

- Administer with food to minimize gastric irritation.
- Advise the patient to take medication exactly as directed. Abrupt withdrawal may cause insomnia, irritability and sometimes even seizures.
- Explain about adverse effects and advise him to avoid activities that require alertness.
- Caution the patient to avoid alcohol or any other CNS depressants along with benzodiazepines.
- If IM administration is preferred give deep IM.
- For IV administration do not mix with any other drugs. Give slow IV as respiratory or cardiac arrest can occur: Monitor vital signs during IV administration.

Chapter 5

Sedatives and Hypnotics

INTRODUCTION

It is rapidly emerging as a first line drug for treatment of mania.

Valproic acid was first synthesized by Burton and used as organic solvent. It was approved by US FDA as an antiepileptic drug for absence seizures in 1978 and for the treatment of acute mania in 1996.

The term valproate is often used to denote all commercial preparations since the common entity in blood is valproic acid.

1. Valproate sodium
2. Divalproex
3. Chrono preparation.

INDICATION

- Acute mania, prophylactic treatment of bipolar-I disorder, rapid cycling bipolar disorder.
  - Schizoaffective disorder
  - Other disorders like bulimia, nervosa, obsessive-compulsive disorder, agitation and PTSD.

Bipolar Disorder

i. *Acute Mania* (as a first line agent for R_x of acute mania in oral and IV forms) several factors associated with a favorable antimanic response to valproate (as well as carbamazepine).
   a. Comorbid substance abuse.
   b. Late age of onset and shorter duration of illness.
   c. History of poor response to lithium dysphoric mania, mixed affective episodes, and rapid cycling.
   d. Organic/complicated mania associated with seizure disorder, and head trauma.
   e. D–M–I (Depression-Mania–Well Interval).

ii. *Prophylaxis* valproate is less effective in the maintenance treatment of bipolar disorder than in treatment of acute mania. It has been used alone as well as long with lithium and other mood stabilizers in maintenance treatment.

iii. *Rapid cycling bipolar disorders and mixed/dysphoric mania*: Patients with rapid cycling mixed affective episodes or dysphoric mania are often resistant to lithium treatment and respond better to valproate.
iv. *Bipolar depression*: Valproate appears to be more effective in the R_x of acute mania than in depression.

Neurological Disorders

i. *Migraine and pain syndrome*: Valproate has been used for the prophylaxis of migraine headaches, as well as for aborting an acute attack also used in trigeminal neuralgia and neuropathic pain.
ii. *Seizure disorder*: Valproate is primarily indicated for R_x of absence seizures, complex partial seizures, myoclonic seizures generalized tonic-clonic seizures.

Other Disorders

Also been used in behavioral afitation in dementia, severe behaviroal symptoms in mental retardation, schizoaffective disorder, alcohol withdrawal, tardive dyskinesia, impulse control disorder, and panic disorder.

SIDE EFFECTS

Nausea, sedation, tremor, flushing, weight gain, thrombocytopenia, menstrual disturbance (in women), and hair loss. There are some reports of polycystic ovaries and hyperandrogenism in young women with epilepsy.

Serious side effect are hepatic toxicity acute hemorrhagic pancreatitis. Use of valproate in pregnancy and lactation should be avoided.

DRUG INTERACTION

Certain drug may increase (e.g. Aspirin, cimetidine ibuprofen, erythromycin, and fluoxitine) or decrease (carbamazepine, phenytoin, phenobarbital refampicin) the serum levels of valproate, valproate increase levels of other drugs (e.g. Lamoteifine, and tricyclic antidepressants).

MECHANISM OF ACTION

The drug acts on gamma-aminobutyric acid [GABA] an inhibitory amino acid neurotransmitter. GABA receptor activation serves to reduce neuronal excitability.

DOSAGE

The usual dose is 15 mg/kg/day with a maximum of 60 mg/kg/day orally.

SIDE EFFECTS

- Nausea, vomiting, and diarrhea.
- Sedation, ataxia, dysarthria, tremor, weight gain, and loss of hair. Thrombocytopenia, and platelet dysfunction.

Nausea, sedation, tremor, flushing, weight gain, thrombocytopenia, menstrual disturbance (in women), and hair loss. There are some reports of polycystic ovaries and hyperandrogenism in young women with epilepsy.

Serious side effects are hepatic toxicity and acute hemorrhagic pancreatitis. Use of valproate in pregnancy and lactation should be avoided.

NURSE'S RESPONSIBILITIES

- Advise the patient to take the drug immediately after food to reduce GI irritation.
- Advise regular follow-up, and periodic examination of blood count, hepatic function and thyroid function.
- Therapeutic serum level of valproic acid is 50 mg – 100 mg/ml.

Chapter 6

Antiparkinsonism Agents

INTRODUCTION

In clinical practice anticholinergic drugs, amitadine and the antihistamines have their primary use as treatments for medication-induced movement disorders, particularly neuroleptic-induced parkinsonism, acute dystonia, and medication-induced tremor.

Anticholinergics – Trihexyphenidyl
– Benztropine
– Biperiden.

Dopaminergic Agents – Bromocriptine
– Carbidopa/ Levodopa

Monoamine Oxidase Type B inhibitors–

- Selegiline

Trihexyphenidyl (Artane, trihexane, trihexy, and pacitane).

INDICATIONS

1. Drug-induced parkinsonism
2. Adjunct in the management of parkinsonism.

MECHANISM OF ACTION

It acts by increasing the release of dopamine from presynaptic vesicles, blocking the reuptake of dopamine into presynaptic nerve terminals or by exerting an agonist defect on postsynaptic dopamine receptors. Trihexyphenidyl reaches peak plasma concentrations in 2–3 hours after oral administration and has duration of action upto 12 hours.

DOSAGE

1 mg – 2 mg per day orally initially, maximum dose upto 15 mg/day in divided doses.

SIDE EFFECTS

- Dizziness, and nervousness
- Drowsiness, weakness, and headache

- Confusion, and blurred vision
- Mydriasis, and tachycardia
- Orthostatic hypotension
- Dry mouth, nausea, and constipation
- Vomiting
- Urinary retention and decreased sweating.

NURSE'S RESPONSIBILITIES

- Assess parkinsonism and extrapyramidal symptoms.
- Medication should be tapered gradually.
- Caution, patient to make position changes slowly to minimize orthostatic hypotension.
- Instruct the patient about frequent rinsing of mouth and good oral hygiene.
- Caution, the patient when this medication decreases, perspiration, and overheating may occur during hot weather.

Chapter 7 Antabuse Drugs

INTRODUCTION

Disulfiram is an important drug in this class and is used to ensure abstinence in the treatment of alcohol dependence. Its main effect is to produce a rapid and violently unpleasant reaction in a person who ingests even a small amount of alcohol while taking disulfiram.

Antabuse has been used since 1951 to help people stop drinking (the generic name of antabuse is Disulfiram). Antabuse is not only effective for stopping drinking. If you have a drug problem, anything that helps you stop drinking will also help you stop using drugs, because alcohol usually leads to drugs.

Antabuse works by making you sick to your stomach if you have a drink. It works because if you know you can't drink, then you won't think about drinking as much.

Numerous studies have proven that antabuse is effective. It has been shown to reduce cravings for alcohol and to reduce the risk of relapse. It has also proven to reduce the risk of relapse in adolescent addicts.

People who use antabuse feel liberated. That internal struggle that goes on everyday, 'Will I drink? Won't I drink?' Is silenced when you're on antabuse. Because drinking is not an option you don't waste your time thinking about drinking, and instead you focus more on your recovery.

Antabuse is effective, because you have to wait for one to two weeks before you can have a drink after you stop antabuse. You can't stop antabuse one day and have a drink the next. It gives you plenty of time to reconsider, restart your antabuse, and ask for help.

Antabuse is a bridge between your two lives. On the one hand, you have the life that you know. It's not what's good for you, but it's what you know. On the other hand, you have the life that you want to get to. It's better for you, but you don't know how to live there. You don't know how to relax, reward yourself, and celebrate without using drugs or alcohol. Antabuse helps you live in that lifelong enough, so that you can develop new habits and coping skills.

DEFINITION

Antabuse, or disulfiram as it is also known, was the first medicine approved for the treatment of alcohol abuse and alcohol-dependence by the US. Food and Drug Administration.

Antabuse is prescribed to help people who want to quit drinking by causing a negative reaction if the person drinks while they are taking antabuse.

MECHANISM OF ACTION

When alcohol is consumed it is metabolized by the body into acetaldehyde, a very toxic substance that causes many hangover symptoms heavy drinkers experience. Usually, the body continues to oxidize acetaldehyde into acetic acid, which is harmless.

Antabuse interferes with this metabolic process, stops the process with the production of acetaldehyde and prevents the oxidation of acetaldehyde into acetic acid. Because of this, antabuse will cause a build up of acetaldehyde 5 or 10 times greater than normally occurs when someone drinks alcohol.

ANTABUSE REACTION

It takes one drink to produce a reaction. It takes one bottle of beer, one glass of wine, or one shot of liquor to become sick.

The normal sequence of the antabuse reaction is—

- Flushing of the face
- Headache
- Low blood pressure
- Racing heart
- Dizziness
- Nausea and vomiting.

If you have one drink, you will vomit about as much as if you had food poisoning.

A few people are very sensitive to antabuse and get a stronger reaction. A quick test of whether you're sensitive to antabuse is to see if your skin flushes when you put alcohol on your skin. If you're sensitive, you may still decide to use antabuse, but you'll have to be a little more careful about avoiding alcohol. Most people just need to show some common sense when they're on antabuse.

EFFECT OF ANTABUSE

The high concentration of acetaldehyde that occurs when someone drinks while taking antabuse can cause reactions that range widely from mild to severe, depending on how much antabuse and how much alcohol is consumed, none of which are pleasant.

If you drink while taking **antabuse**, you can experience these symptoms:

- Flushing
- Nausea
- Copious vomiting
- Sweating
- Thirst
- Throbbing in the head and neck
- Throbbing headache
- Respiratory difficulty
- Chest pain
- Palpitations
- Dyspnea
- Hyperventilation
- Tachycardia
- Hypotension
- Syncope
- Marked uneasiness
- Weakness
- Vertigo
- Blurred vision
- Confusion.

Those are the 'mild' symptoms. Severe reactions can include respiratory depression, cardiovascular collapse, myocardial infarction, acute congestive heart failure, unconsciousness, arrhythmias, convulsions, and death.

USE OF ANTABUSE

Only someone who wants to try to quit drinking and who is fully aware of the consequences of drinking while on the medication should take antabuse. Antabuse should never be given to some without their full knowledge or to anyone who is intoxicated.

Because of the possible severe reactions, antabuse should not be given to anyone with a history of severe heart disease, psychosis, or an allergy to antabuse. Women who are pregnant should not take antabuse and no one taking paraldehyde or metronidazole should use antabuse.

ANTABUSE DOES NOT DO

Antabuse serves merely as physical and psychological deterrent to someone trying to stop drinking. It does not reduce the person's craving for alcohol, nor does it treat any **alcohol withdrawal symptoms**.

DO'S AND DON'TS OF ANTABUSE

Wait at least 24 hours after drinking before starting antabuse. Consider the following arithmetic. If you had 10 drinks and weighed only 100 Ibs (45 kg), the alcohol would be completely eliminated from your system in 24 hours. If you weighed more than 100 Ibs (45 kg) it would take less than 24 hours.

For most people, it takes one drink to produce an antabuse reaction, therefore it's hard to get by mistake. You can have foods that have been cooked in wine, as long as they've been cooked the alcohol evaporates quickly. You have to be careful of some deserts that have a lot of uncooked alcohol in them. You also have to be careful of some cough syrups and cold preparations that can contain as much as 40% alcohol.

Most people prefer to use nonalcoholic mouthwashes to be on the safe side. Although the amount of alcohol you absorb from mouthwash does'nt equal one drink, assuming you don't drink your mouthwash.

You can use perfumes, colognes, or aftershaves. The amount of alcohol you absorb through your skin is minimal.

The standard patient information sheet on antabuse says that you should avoid all of these things: Mouthwash, perfumes, colognes, even vinegar. But I've treated thousands of patients, and I've never known any of them to get a reaction from anything other than drinking. Antabuse liberates you, if you use a little common sense.

EFFECTIVENESS OF ANTABUSE

The effectiveness of antabuse in helping someone quit drinking depends on the person's continued use of medication. Because antabuse is administered in a daily pill, people can merely stop taking the drug and begin drinking a few days later.

However, research in Europe, where antabuse is much more widely used than in the United States, has shown that **long-term use of antabuse is very effective** in helping people stop drinking, producing abstinence rates of 50 percent. The longer people take antabuse, the more effective it is, because they develop a 'habit' of not drinking, research revealed.

SIDE EFFECTS

The side effects of antabuse are less common than the side effects of relapse. During the first week or two that you take antabuse, you'll probably feel a little more tired. It usually lasts for a week or two and then it goes away.

During the first two months that people take antabuse, about 20% develop a funny taste in their mouth. It's usually decribed as a metallic taste. Eighty percent of people don't get it, and if you do get that taste, it often goes away after a few weeks or months. That's it for the minor side effects of antabuse.

The major side effects of antabuse are rare. The most common but still rare side effect of antabuse is liver damage. Any drug that you take over a long-term has the potential to cause liver damage. With antabuse, it happens in roughly one out of 30,000 people.

Your doctor can do a simple blood test to check the state of your liver before you start. After you've been on antabuse for a month you should have your liver tests repeated. Your doctor should periodically check your liver enzymes while you're on antabuse.

Any drug can have any possible side effect. You can never say never in medicine. Every year people die from taking tylenol (acetaminophen). But that doesn't mean we should stop using tylenol. The benefits far outweigh the risks. And the benefits of antabuse outweigh the risks of drinking.

Before taking antabuse you should give your doctor your entire medical history. You may not be able to take antabuse if you have a significant medical history of heart or blood vessel disease, diabetes, and underactive thyroid, brain disorders (e.g. seizures, brain damage), kidney disease, liver disease, a history of severe depression, a history of psychosis, or a history of suicide attempts. Antabuse can alter the metabolism and blood levels of certain drugs, especially tricyclic antidepressants, Dilantin (phenytoin), coumadin, isoniazid, and theophyline.

Do not take antabuse if you're pregnant, or trying to become pregnant.

SERIOUS WARNING SIGNS

If you notice any of the following rare but serious warning signs, stop using antabuse and tell your doctor immediately: Dark urine, severe abdominal pain, presistent nausea or vomiting, and yellowing of the eyes or skin.

RESISTANCE TO TRYING ANTABUSE

There are only three reasons why you may be reluctant to try antabuse.

First, because you're worried about the side effects. Although the side effects of antabuse can be serious, they are rare. The side effects of relapsing on alcohol are common and serious.

The second reason is because you want to do your recovery on your own. You've always been self-reliant and you want to be self-reliant in your recovery. But recovery involves learning to ask for help. Doing it on your own is overrated. You need to ask for help from your doctor, treatment program, 12 step group, and sponsor. Antabuse is just one more thing you can use. It is not an alternative to your supports. It complements them.

The third and final reason why you may be reluctant to try antabuse is because you want to leave the door open to having a drink. Just in case you want to relapse there won't be anything in your way. Of course, if you leave that door open then it's guaranteed you'll relapse eventually. It's just a matter of time.

If you've decided that you want to change your life. If you've decided that you have suffered enough negative consequences, then I encourage you to talk to your doctor about antabuse.

GETTING A PRESCRIPTION

Speak to your doctor about antabuse. Antabuse is available at most pharmacies, and is a simple drug that can be made by most pharmacists. If you are a Canadian resident and your doctor cannot find a pharmacy that dispenses antabuse, it can be ordered through *www.pharmacy.ca*, which is an internet pharmacy that delivers free of charge through Canada Post.

ANTIALCOHOL DRUGS

There are three antialcohol drugs available:

- Antabuse (disulfiram)
- Campral (acamprosate)
- Revia (naltrexone).

I have focused on antabuse for a few reasons. It has a long track record, and is considered safe and effective. Its available in generic form, which means that it's quite inexpensive. The cost of antabuse is a lot less than the price of alcohol.

Studies have shown that antabuse is at least as effective, and sometime more effective than the other two medications, which have only been around for a few years 5–6 years.

A RECOVERY CHECKLIST

A list of important goals for the first year of your recovery. Use it as a reminder and to help you stay on track in the days and months ahead.

- Accept that you have and addiction
- Practice honesty in your life
- Learn to avoid high-risk situations
- Ask for help
- Practice calling friends before you have cravings
- Become actively involved in self-help recovery groups
- Go to discussion meetings and begin to share
- Get a sponsor and do step work
- Get rid of using friends
- Make time for you and your recovery
- Celebrate your small victories. Recovery is about progress not perfection
- Practice saying no
- Take better care of yourself
- Develop healthy eating and sleeping habits
- Learn to relax and let go of stress
- Discover how to have fun, clean and sober
- Make new recovery friends and bring them into your life
- 'Play the tape forward' to deal with cravings
- Find ways to distract yourself when you have cravings

- Deal with postacute withdrawal symptoms
- Develop a strategy for social settings where drinking is involved
- Thank the supportive people in your life
- Develop tolerance and compassion for yourself and others
- Say goodbye to your addiction
- See yourself as a nonuser.

HELP FOR THE FAMILY

An addiction destroys families as much as it destroys individuals. Living with an addict is both heartbreaking and exhausting. Family members are torn between how to help the addict and how to avoid being sucked into the addict's world.

Here are some helpful suggestions that I have found over the years of working with addicts and their families. I hope they can help you.

THINGS YOU CAN DO FOR THE ADDICT

- Behave exactly as you would if your loved one had a serious illness. What would you do if they were diagnosed with heart disease or cancer?
- Educate yourself on addiction and recovery.
- Try not to accuse or judge. Avoid name calling. This is a difficult time for both of you.
- Provide a sober environment that reduces triggers for using.
- Allow the addict time to go to meetings.
- Understand that your lives will change. Do not wish for your old life back. Your old life to some extent is what got you here. You both need to create a new life where it is easier to not use alcohol or drugs.
- Make sure that you both have time for fun. People use alcohol and drugs to relax, escape, and as a reward. The addict needs to find alternative ways to relax, escape, and as a reward otherwise they will turn back to their addiction.
- Do not enable. Do not provide excuse or cover up for the addict.
- Do not shield the addict from the consequences of their addiction. People are more likely to change if they have suffered enough negative consequences.
- Set boundaries that you all agree on. The goal of boundaries is to improve the health of the family as a whole. Do not use boundaries to punish or shame.
- If you want to provide financial support, buy the goods and services the addict needs instead of giving them money that they might use to buy alcohol or drugs.
- Recognize and acknowledge the potential the addict has within them.

THINGS YOU CAN DO FOR YOURSELF

- Take care of yourself. Living with an addict is exausting. You also need time to recover.
- Avoid self-blame. You can't control another person's decisions, and you can't force them to change.
- Do not work harder than the addict. The best approach is not to do things for the addict, but instead to be an example of balance and self-care.
- Being a caretaker is not good for you or the addict. Understand that there is only so much you can do to change another person.
- Ask for help. Talk to professional. Go to a support group such as Al-Anon. (More support groups are listed below).
- Do not argue or try to discuss things with the addict when they are under the influence. It won't get you anywhere.
- If at all possible, try not to be negative when dealing with the addict. That may only increase their feelings of guilt and push them further into using.

THE THREE C'S OF DEALING WITH AN ADDICT

- You didn't cause the addiction
- You can't control the addiction
- You can't cure the addiction.

'**You can't stop drinking or using for another person**'.

HELPFUL LINKS FOR FAMILY AND FRIENDS OF ADDICTS

- Al-Anon.org (al-anon.org) for family members of alcoholics
- Nar-anon (nar-anon.org) for family members of addicts
- Gam-anon (gam-anon.org) for family members of gamblers
- Coda.org (coda.org) for co-dependent individuals
- Adultchildren.org (adultchildren.org) for adult children of alcoholics and addicts.

12 STEP GROUPS

- Alcoholics Anonymous (AA) (aa.org)
- Adult Children of Alcoholics (ACA) (adultchild.org)
- All-Addictions Anonymous (alladdictionsanonymous.com)
- Al-Anon.org (al-anon.org) for family members of addicts
- Cocaine Anonymous (CA) (ca.org)
- Crystal Meth Anonymous (CMA) (crystameth.org)
- Dual Recovery Anonymous (UK): A 12-setp Program for those with a dual diagnosis
- Food Addicts in Recovery Anonymous (FA) (foodaddicts.org)
- Gamblers Anonymous (GA) (gamblersanonymous.org)

- Narcotics Anonymous (NA) (na.org)
- Nar-Anon (nar-anon.org) for family members of addicts
- Nicotine Anonymous (nicotine-anonymous.org)
- Marijuana Anonymous (marijuana-anonymous.org)
- Methadone Anonymous (methadoneanonymous.info)
- S-Anon (sanon.org)
- Sex and Love Addicts Anonymous (SLAA) (slaafws.org)
- Women for Sobriety (WFS) (womenforsobriety.org)
- XA Speakers (xa-speakers.org) A collection of recordings from speaker meetings, conventions and workshops of 12-step groups.
- 12 Steps (12step.org) Resources for all 12 step programs. It contains an in-depth discussion and forum on the 12 steps.
- 12StepTreatmentCenters.com A list of 12 Step treatment centers around the world.

GOVERNMENT AGENCIES

- National Institute of Alcohol Abuse and Alcoholism (niaaa.nih.gov)
- National Institute of Drug Abuse (nida.nih.gov)
- National Clearinghous for Alcohol and Drug Information (ncadi. samhsa.gov)
- Substance Abuse and Mental Health Services Administration (samhsa.gov)
- National Institute of Mental Health (nimh.nih.gov)
- Smoke Free (smokefree.gov)
- World Health Organization.

ORGANIZATIONS

- Addiction Recovery Guide Addiction and recovery resources
- American Lung Association (lungusa.org)
- American Society of Addiction Medicine (asam.org)
- Benzodiazepine Addiction, Withdrawal and Recovery (benzo.org.uk)
- Canadian Addiction, Counsellors Certification Federation (caccf.ca). An organization that certifies and monitors addiction counselors in Canada.
- Canadian Lung Association (lung. ca)
- Canadian Society of Addiction Medicine (csam.org)
- Employee Assistance Professionals Association (eapassn. org)
- Employee Assistance Program Association of Toronto (eapat.org)
- Helping Others Live Sober Aimed at people in recovery and professionals. Together, we are united in the shared goal of Helping Others Live Sober.
- International Center for Alcohol Policies (icap.org)
- National Association of Alcoholism and Drug Abuse Counselors (NAADAC) (naadac.org) An organization that certifies and monitors addiction counselors.

- Partnership for Drug Free America(drugfree.org)
- Project Cork (projectcork.org).

OTHER RESOURCES

- AddictionsSearch.com
- Alcohol Rehab
- Bellwood
- Benzo Withdrawal Forums Online group for benzodiazepine addiction, withdrawal and recovery.(benzowithdrawal.org)
- Crossorads (Antigua)
- Drug and Alcohol Treatment Referral
- Food Addiction
- Metamorphosis Clinic
- My Addiction
- Overcoming Addiction
- Pressing The Issue
- Stop And Think Radio
- Recovery Connection
- Support Groups
- Valley Hope: Drug and alcohol rehab nonprofit organization.

ADDICTION TEST

Answer the following seven yes or no questions. Most questions have more than one part, because everyone behaves differently in addiction. You only need to answer yes to one part for that question to count as a positive response.

1. **Tolerance**: Has your use of drugs or alcohol increased over time?
2. **Withdrawal**: When you stop using, have you ever experienced physical or emotional withdrawal? Have you had any of the following symptoms: Irritability, anxiety, shakes, sweats, nausea, or vomiting?
3. **Difficulty controlling your use**: Do you sometimes use more or for a longer time than you would like? Do you sometimes drink to get drunk? Do you stop after a few drink usually, or does one drink lead to more drinks?
4. **Negative consequences**: Have you continued to use even though there have been negative consequences to your mood, self-esteem, health, job, or family?
5. **Putting off or neglecting activities**: Have you ever put off or reduced social, recreational, work, or household activities because of your use?
6. **Spending significant time or emotional energy**: Have you spent a significant amount of time obtaining, using, concealing, planning, or recovering from your use? Have you spend a lot of time thinking about using? Have you ever concealed or minimized your use? Have you ever thought of schemes to avoid getting caught?

7. **Desire to cut down**: Have you sometimes thought about cutting down or controlling your use? Have you ever made unsuccessful attempts to cut down or control your use?

If you answered yes to at least 3 of these questions, then you meet the medical criteria (DSM and ICD) for addiction.

There are no restrictions on the printing of this document. It is provided as a public service by www.AddictionAndRecovery.org. For a more complete guide to addiction refer to the book 'I Want to Change My Life' by Dr. Steven M. Melemis.

DEPRESSION TEST

Answer the following 10 yes or no questions. Most questions have more than one part, because everyone feels their depression differently. You need to answer yes to only one part per question in order for that question to count.

1. **Depressed mood**: Do you feel sad, down, or depressed most of the time? Do you feel that all the color has been drained out of your life? Do you cry more easily? Do you have crying spells for no apparent reason?
2. **Loss of interest**: Have you lost interest in things that used to give you enjoyment? Have you lost interest or enjoyment in the activities of daily life? Are you more socially withdrawn or isolated?
3. **Low energy**: Is your energy lower? Do you feel more fatigued or sluggish? Is it hard to get going in the morning? Is your libido suddenly reduced or do you have less interest in sex?
4. **Anxiety or irritability**: Are you more anxious, worried, fearful, irritable, or intolerant?
5. **Lower self-confidence**: Is your self-confidence or self-esteem lower? Do you feel more hopeless or pessimistic? Do you feel more guilty or worthless?
6. **Poor concentration**: Is it hard for you to think, concentrate, or make decisions? Do you find it hard to concentrate outside of work? Do you find it harder to read articles or to take in what you read?
7. **Sleep changes**: Do you have difficulty falling asleep or staying asleep? On the weekends do you feel like you could sleep all day and don't want to get out of bed? Do you feel that you're not refreshed when you wake up in the morning?
8. **Appetite or weight change**: Is your appetite either significantly lower or higher than a year ago? Have you unintentionally lost or gained weight? Do you eat only because you have to eat, but don't get any pleasure from food?
9. **Slow moving or restless**: Are you more slow moving lately? Is your speech slower lately? Do you feel like you're shuffling when you walk? Are you restless or fidgety? Do you wring your hands more?

10. **Thoughts of death**: Do you have recurrent thoughts of death or suicide (not just a fear of dying)? Do you think it would be easier if you just didn't wake up in the morning? Do you think it would be easier if you developed a serious illness? Do you wonder if anyone will miss you when you're gone? Do you think you would be better off dead, or that your family would be better off if you were gone? Do you imagine ways of hurting yourself?

If you answered yes to at least 5 of these questions, then you meet the medical criteria (DSM and ICD) for depression.

There are no restrictions on the printing of this document. It is provided as a public service by www.AnxietyDepressionHealth.org. For a more complete guide to depression refer to the book 'I Want to Change My Life' by Dr. Steven M. Melemis.

Chapter 8

Drugs Used in Child Psychiatry

CLONIDINE

Indications

Control of withdrawal symptoms from opioids
- Tourette's disorders
- Control of aggressive or hyperactive behavior in children
- Autism.

Mechanism of Action

- Alpha 2- adrenergic receptor agonist
- The agonist effects of clonidine on presynaptic alpha 2-adrenergic receptors result in a decrease in the amount of neurotransmitter released from the presynaptic nerve terminal.

Dosage

Usual starting dosage is 0.1 mg orally twice a day: The dosage can be raised by 0.3 mg a day to an appropriate level.

Side Effects

- Dry mouth, dryness of eyes, and fatigue
- Irritability and sedation
- Dizziness, nausea, and vomiting
- Hypotension and constipation.

Nurse's Responsibilities

- Monitor BP, the drug should be withheld if the patient becomes hypotensive.
- Advise frequent mouth rinses and good oral hygiene for dry mouth.

METHYLPHENIDATE [RITALIN]

Methylphenidate, dextroamphetamine and pemoline are sympathomimetics.

Indications

- Attention-deficit hyperactivity disorder
- Narcolepsy
- Depressive disorders
- Obesity.

Mechanism of Action

- Sympathomimetics cause the stimulation of alpha and beta-adrenergic receptors directly as agonists and indirectly by stimulating the release of dopamine and norepinephrine from presynaptic terminals.
- Dextroamphetamine and methylphenidate are also inhibitors of catecholamine reuptake, especially dopamine reuptake and inhibitors of monoamino oxidase. The next result of these activities is believed to be the stimulation of several brain regions.

Dosage

Starting dose is 5 mg – 10 mg per day orally, maximum daily dose is 80 mg/day.

Side Effects

- Anorexia or dyspepsia
- Weight loss, slowed growth
- Dizziness
- Insomnia or nightmares
- Dysphoric mood, tics and psychosis.

Nurse's Responsibilities

- Assess mental status for change in mood, level of activity, degree of stimulation, and aggressiveness.
- Ensure that patient is protected from injury.
- Keep stimuli low and environment as quick as possible to discourage overstimulation.
- To decrease anorexia, the medication may be administered immediately after meal.
- The patient should be weighted regularly during hospitalization.
- To prevent insomnia administer last dose at least 6 hours before bedtime.
- In children with behavior disorders a drug 'holiday' should be attempted periodically under the direction of the physician to determine effectiveness of the medication and the need for continuation.
- Ensure that parents are aware of the delayed effects of Ritalin. Therapeutic response may not be seen for 2–4 weeks, the drugs should not be discontinued for lack of immediate results.

- Inform patients that OTC (over-the-counter) medications should be avoided while the child is on stimulant medication.
- Some OTC medications, particularly cold and hay fever preparations contain certain sympathomimetic agents that could compound the effect of the stimulant and create drug interactions that may be toxic to the child.
- Ensure that parents are aware that the drug should not be withdrawn abrupt.

BIBLIOGRAPHY

1. Sreevani R. A Guide to Mental Health and Psychiatric Nursing; 3rd ed. Jaypee Brothers Medical Publishers(P) Ltd: New Delhi. 2009; 93 – 106.

UNIT-II
Psychological Therapies

- Individual Psychotherapy
- Group Pschotherapy and Supportive Psychotherapy
- Family Therapy
- Behavior Therapy
- Hypnosis or Hypnotherapy
- Narcoanalysis
- Milieu Therapy
- Therapeutic Community

INTRODUCTION

Psychotherapy is defined as a treatment for problems of an emotional nature in which a trained person deliberately establishes a professional relationship with the patient to remove, modified or retarded existing symptoms, disturbed pattern of behavior and promote positive personality growth and development.

DEFINITION OF PSYCHOTHERAPY

According to Lego S. defines psychotherapy—'A method of treatment based on the development of therapeutic relationship between client and therapist for the purpose of exploring and modifying the patient's behavior in a satisfying direction'.

CONCEPT OF PSYCHOTHERAPY

1. A therapeutic relationship is established between the patient and the therapist.
2. To modify, remove or reduce the factors causing a disturbed behavior.

3. To help the patient to grow and develop coping mechanism to face the problem in future and improve in social functioning.

GOALS OF PSYCHOTHERAPY

1. Changing maladaptive behavior
2. Modifying environment causing maladaptive behavior
3. Improving IPR skills
4. Helping the patient to overcome a feeling of handicap
5. Helping him to make an accurate assessment of himself and develop self-identity.

TYPES AND TECHNIQUES OF PSYCHOTHERAPY

Psychotherapy

1) Individual psychotherapy	2) Behavioral psychotherapy	3) Interpersonal psychotherapy	4) Group psychotherapy
• Psychoanalysis	• Behavior modification	• Marital therapy	
• Hypnosis	• Systematic desensitization	• Family therapy	
• Narcoanalysis			
• Abreaction	• Aversion therapy	• Transactional therapy	
• Reality therapy	• Assertive training		
• Uncovering	• Cognitive behavior therapy		
• **Supportive psychotherapy** ↓			
1. Ventilation	• Implosive therapy or flooding		
2. Environmental modification			
3. Persuasion	• Positive reinforcement		
4. Re-education	• Response shaping		
5. Reassurance	• Modeling		
	• Token economy		

CONTRAINDICATIONS

- Psychotic patient with severe behavior disturbance like excitement
- Organic psychosis, hysteria, and personality disorder (malingering)
- Patient who are unmotivated and unwilling to accept it.

Chapter 9 Individual Psychotherapy

INTRODUCTION

It is conducted on a one-to-one basis, i.e. the therapist treats one client at a time. The patient is encouraged to discover for himself the reason for his behavior. The therapist listens to the patient and offers explanation and advice when necessary.

OVERVIEW

Psychotherapy is the use of technique that facilitates or allows people to modify their feelings attitudes and behaviors. Individual psychotherapy focuses on the needs and problems of the client. In therapy two people come together in an encounter that is specifically designed for the purposes of relieving emotional pain, treating mental illness and facilitating change and growth. In a therapy situation one person is designates as therapist (the facilitating and helping person) and the other is called client and therapist will discuss some historical information, current challenges, past success, feelings, needs, and goals. Because of their objectivity and specialized knowledge, therapist can be generally more effective than family or friends in facilitating the client's with challenges and growth.

DEFINITION

Psychotherapy conducted on a one-to-one setting. These techniques are designed to help persons overcome mental distress and illness for the purpose of assisting the individual to reach their optimum level of health the effectiveness of such therapy depend on the patient-therapist relationship.

APPROACHES TO INDIVIDUAL PSYCHOTHERAPY

These are multiple approaches to therapy:

1. Insight oriented therapy—It derives from psychoanalysis for helping the individual to gain insight into feelings and behavior. In this, the therapist try to bring out the unconscious conflicts and feelings that

causes anxiety into the conscious level. Insight therapy uses exploring and giving meaning to irrational feeling and maladaptations.

2. Task-oriented therapy—This will help to gain tool that will help them to change their behavior.
3. Experience-oriented—These attempt will increased on experience that will help growth and personality development.

LEVELS OF INDIVIDUAL PSYCHOTHERAPY

1. *Supportive*: The client is providing the caring, safe relationship in which to explore problems make decisions. The therapist reinforces client's existing coping skills and does not attempt to teach him/her new coping methods.
2. *Re-educative*: The clients explore new way to perceive and behave through a systematic approach. The client and therapist sign a contract that identifies goals and desired changes in behaviors and feelings. An effective approach is reality-based focused on solutions and directly deals with concrete issues. Examples include cognitive restructuring and behavior modification.
3. *Reconstructive*: The client may spend two to five years exploring all aspects of his/her life through analysis or deep psychotherapy. Outcomes include self-understanding and understanding of others greater emotional freedom, maximizing one's potentials, and greater capacity for love and work.

Indications

- Stress-related disorders
- Alcohol and drug dependence
- Sexual disorders
- Marital disharmony.

PROCESS OF PSYCHOTHERAPY (FIG. 9.1)

Assessment—It serves as a basis for developing plan of care and gives clients baseline to measure his/her progress.

Planning—Plan of care is negotiated among client, nurses, family and health care team. Identifies expected outcomes and set a goals.

Goals

Two types of goals are—

Long-term goal	*Short-term goal*
Prevention of recurrence discharge planning	Relief from immediate problem

Implementation—Provides psychotherapy on one-to-one basis or to individual, group and families.

Evaluation—Identifies client's progress in attaining expected outcomes.

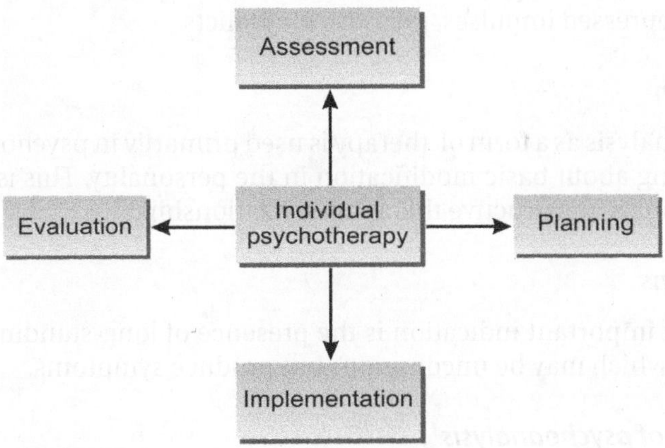

Figure.9.1: Process of psychotherapy

STAGES OF INDIVIDUAL PSYCHOTHERAPY

There are mainly three stages of individual psychotherapy.

Introductory Stage

The client and therapist meet and begin to work together. This stage usually involves taking a history of the client's life including medical problems and current medications if the client is a referral. The therapist may already have the information.

The introductory phase completed in 6, 10 or 20 sessions.

Working Stage

The client is able to become more trusting to disclose and to begin exploring with the therapist the thoughts, feelings, and behavior that lead to pain or problems. The whole process may be completed in 20 sessions. As the client understands and functions more effectively the last stage of working through is reached.

Working Through Stage

The client achieved higher level of understanding or the self and relationship with others and begins to tryout new ways of perceiving, thinking, feeling, and behaving. As the client interacts with others and see newly acquired coping skills.

TYPES OF INDIVIDUAL PSYCHOTHERAPY

I. Psychoanalysis

Psychoanalysis was first developed by 'Sigmund Freud'. The therapeutic techniques focuses primarily on the influence of unconscious forces such as repressed impulses, memories, conflicts.

Definition

'Psychoanalysis as a form of therapy is used primarily in psychoneuroses by bringing about basic modification in the personality. This is done by establishing a constructive therapeutic relationship.'

Indications

The most important indication is the presence of long-standing mental conflicts which may be unconscious but produce symptoms.

Methods of psychoanalysis

The specific methods are free association, dream interpretation. Analysis of resistances and defences used by the patient, working through the feelings and experiences revealed by the patient during transference.

1. *Free association*—It refers to the verbalization of thoughts as they occur, without any conscious screening. It is make use of that to affect reconstruction of personality.

2. *Dream interpretation*—Analysis of dream helps to gain additional insight into his problems the resistances. Thus dreams symbolically communicate areas of intrapsychic conflict.

3. *Transference reaction*—It refers to the patient's development of strong positive or negative feelings towards of the analyst and they represent the patient's past response.

Process of psychoanalysis

1. The role of the patient and psychoanalyst are explicity defined by Freud.
2. The patient is an active participant, freely revealing all thoughts exactly as they occur and describing all dreams.
3. He is frequently in a recumbent position on a couch during therapy to induce relaxation, which facilitates free association.
4. The psychoanalyst is a shadow person. He reveals nothing personal, nor does he gives any direction to the patient. His verbal response is most brief and not interfere with the associative flow.
5. He depacts from this style of communication when an interpretation of behavior is made to the patient.

6. By termination of therapy, the patient is able to conduct his life according to an accurate assessment of external reality.
7. It is a long-term proposition. Every interaction for 45 minutes, 4 to 5 days a weeks for approx 3 to 5 years.
8. It is an expensive and time-consuming therapy.

Types of psychoanalysis

a. Classical psychoanalysis—Its come under in freudian psychoanalysis, the therapist remain passive and approach is nondirective. He constantly challenges defenses, interprets, transference, and interpretation.

b. Psychoanalytically-oriented psychotherapy—Psychoanalytically-oriented psychotherapy is much more direct form of psychoanalysis. The duration of therapy is briefer and advice is given to the patient occasionally. The patient and therapist sit face to face. However, additional drug treatment can be use.

Its indication both psychoanalysis and psychoanalytically-oriented psychotherapy are not based on any psychiatric diagnosis.

II. Hypnosis

Hypnoanalysis or hypnotherapy is a method used to help the individual talk about feeling and conflicts about which the individual normally may not be aware of and may not talk about.

Definition

'Hypnoanalysis refers to the method used to get the patient express his unconscious conflict under hypnosis.'

Process of hypnotherapy

Hypnosis is a superficial or deep trance (a somnolent state sleep like) resembling sleep. It is induced in a patient by suggestions of relaxation and concentrating attention on a single object. The client becomes highly suggestible, submissive, and abandons control and response to therapist's influence. He can be induced to recall forgotten events, become insensitive to pain, gains relief from tension, anxiety, and other psychological symptoms.

III. Narcoanalysis

Refers to the method used to help the patient talk under the influence of definite level of narcotic drug given intravenously.

IV. Abreaction

It is a therapeutic technique in which the patient talk about repressed emotions by receiving and relieving painful experiences that have been buried in the unconscious. When the psychiatrist considers that it could be helpful, he may use an intervenous injection of a drug such as pentothal.

V. Reality Therapy

Reality therapy concentrates on the 'here' and 'now' of the behavior. William Glassec explains that the basic needs of human beings are 'to love' and 'to be loved' and 'to feel worthwhile'.

Definition

'This is a psychotherapeutic technique which focuses on the present behavior and development of a patient's ability to cope with the stresses of reality and take a greater responsibility for the fulfilment of his needs.'

Concept/technique of reality therapy

To achieve the purpose of reality therapy the therapist becomes involved in an active relationship with the patient, rejects his unrealistic behavior and teaches better ways to meet his needs in the real world. The patient needs to be stressed on, that the past cannot be changed. So he must take responsibility of right or wrong actions of the present. This therapy is a special kind of teaching which attempt to accomplish in a relatively short intense period in normal growing up.

VI. Insight Psychotherapy or Uncovering

This technique is used to breakthrough the patient's repressed conflict and traumatic experience to the surface it helps the patient in gaining an insight into his conflict or problem and cope with problems.

VII. Supportive Psychotherapy

Definition

'It is a form of psychological treatment given to patient with chronic and disabling psychiatric condition for whom basic charge is not seen as a realistic goal.'

Goals—
- Support reality testing
- Provide ego support
- Maintain or re-establish usual level of functions.

VIII. Other Psychotherapies

1. Re-educative psychotherapies
2. Reconstructive psychotherapies.

1. Re-educative psychotherapies

Which attempt to teach the individual new pattern of behavior and social functioning.

a. **Client-centered psychotherapy**: It was borrowed from the ideas of Carl Rogees (1952). The main condition include—
   1. Client is experiencing at least a vague incongruence which causes him to be anxious.
   2. The therapist is congruent (or genuine or real).
   3. The therapist is experiencing and accurately sensitive to understanding of client's internal frame of reference.
   4. The client perceives to some minimal degree of realness, the caring and understanding of the therapist.

The following attitudes are deemed to be most important for the success of client-centered therapy.
   i. Genuineness
   ii. Unconditioned positive regard
   iii. Accurate empathy.

b. **Gestalt therapy (Frederick Perls [1893–1970])**: Gestalt theory proposes that the natural course of biological and psychological development of the organism entails a full awareness of physical sensation and psychological needs and the organization of behavior in manner to lead to fulfilment of these needs and an appropriate expression of affect, e.g. hunger leads to eating, anger leads to aggression.

c. **Reality therapy**: It is associated with psychological health by need to love and responsibility.

d. **Rational-Emotive psychotherapy (RET)**: It is developed by Albert-Ellis (1913) who believed that emotional distrubances are the end product of irrational or illogical thinking.

   The main aim of the therapy to identify the patient's irrational ideas and to replace them with more realistic and adaptive ones.

e. **Primal therapy**: Developed by Arther Vivian Janov, it asserts that neurosis is the result of failure to satisfy infantile needs.

   Primal therapy represent a patterened, programed, systematic assault is called unreal self. Therapy is time-consuming and taking up a several months and involve abstinence from alcohol, cigarettes, and drugs.

f. **Existential therapy**: Existentialism seeks to characterize man through its 'dynamic' formulations rather than through its essence.

   It is a philosophy of being nothing in the nothingness for a few it supplies the strength to live virtuously in the midst of despair.

g. **Logotherapy**: Developed by Viktor E. Frankl (1905). The Basic source of discomfort and unhappiness can be traced to their failure to find meaning in their lives.

   Logotherapy stresses on the philosophical or spiritual aspects of men.

h. **Psychodrama**: Moreno (1959), its modern founder, quotes instances when it was used by priests in primitive tribes to cure hysterical and anxiety symptoms. The main principle of psychodrama is **Acting out**. In this while the bringing to the surface of important inner experiences giving the therapist and the patient opportunity to evaluate the situation, the latter being called action.
i. **Transactional analysis**: The analysis of the interaction pattern of the individual is the basis of transactional analysis. Eric Burne (1964) explains that individual interacts mainly at 3 levels adult, parent and child. The dysfunctional interpersonal relationship is the cause of the problem. Thus analysis of the interaction patterns provides insight to the problem and the problems can be solved.
j. **Crises therapy**: It may be defined as transitional period which represent an individual with either an opportunity for personality growth and maturation or the risk of adverse effect with increased vulnerability to subsequent stress. Past maladaptive pattern of problem solving may be repeated during crisis.

2. Reconstructive psychotherapy

Which aim to dismantle and rebuilt a new personality?

a. **Jung's therapy**: Jungian therapy emphasizes the value of patients pursing the products of unconscious fantasy through dream, reveries and artistic creativity.
b. **Adlerian therapy**: It reflects on aggession, in the sense of self-assertion and the will to power takes precedence over sex as the prime move of human behavior.
c. **Klein's therapy**: Focuses on the relationship of the developing infant with other couple. He emphasize the impatience of fantasy in the first two year of life. The infant's love and hate are initially directed toward the mother who represent the child's whole world.

Chapter 10 Group Psychotherapy and Supportive Psychotherapy

GROUP PSYCHOTHERAPY

Introduction

It is a treatment modality in which selected group of client are treated by a qualified group therapist. The goal of group therapy is to alleviate their psychic system, to reduce anxiety and modify behavior in controlled setting.

Definition

Group psychotherapy is a treatment in which carefully selected people who are emotionally ill, meet in a group guided by a trained therapist, and help one another effect personality change.

Overview

The goal is group therapy is to help individual develops more functional and satisfying relationship. When an individual's functional pattern is demonstrated in the group, the task of the group is to assist the members to understand the pattern of interacting within the group and to help clients generalize this information to their lives outside the group.

Types of Group Psychotherapy

Therapy group: Group of persons come together to receive psychotherapy in a group setting.

Traditional group: It includes mainly the patient with mental illness and are from the hospital inpatient department.

Encounter group: It is a form of small group in which an individual learns how his feelings and behavior affect him and other.

Homogenous and heterogenous group: Homogenous group consist of patients with same characteristics like age, sex, race, etc. whereas heterogenous group vary in all these aspects.

Open group and closed group: In open group members may join and leave the group at any time. Closed group have specific number of people, specific time to start and close the group sessions.

Group according to mental illness: Neurotic and psychotic patients are in this group.

Task groups: A group formed to accomplish a specific outcome.

Teaching groups: Focus is to convey knowledge and information to a number of individuals.

Supportive/Therapeutic groups: The concern of these groups is to prevent possible future upset by educating the participants in effective ways of dealing with emotional stress arising from situational or development crises.

Self-help groups: Composed of individuals with a similar problem.

Physical conditions that influence group dynamics:

- **Seating**: It is best when there is no barrier between the members. For example, a circle of chairs is better than chairs set around a table.
- **Size**: Seven or eight members provide a favorable climate for optimal group interaction and relationship development.
- **Membership**: Two types of groups exist— **Open-ended groups** (those in which members leave and others join at any time during the existence of the group) and **Closed-ended groups** (those in which all members join at the time the group is organized and terminated at the end of the designated length of time).

Curative/Therapeutic Factors of Group Therapy (According to Yalom)

- Instillation of hope: Client believes he/she will get better through groups therapy.
- Universality: Client learns that other group members have similar problems and feelings.
- Imparting of information: Client learns didactic information which occurs in a group settings.
- Altruism: Client help each other in the group, resulting in increased self-esteem.
- Corrective recapitulation of the primary family group: Client's family background influences client behavior and client can relieve and correct early conflicts.
- Development of socializing techniques: Client develops social skills in the group.
- Initiative behavior: Client identifies with imitates healthy behavior of group members.
- Interpersonal learning: Client's interpersonal distortions are corrected.
- Group cohesiveness: Client experiences bonding with the group, group norms are protected and positive client's outcome results.
- Catharsis: Group members express feelings, even deep and powerful emotions, and then learn new ways to handle their problems.
- Existential factors: Responsibility, existence, awareness, and mortality and explored.

Contraindications

- Antisocial patients
- Actively suicidal or severely depressed patients
- Patient who are delusional and who may incorporate the group into their delusional system.

Group Size

Optimal group size for group therapy is 8–10 members.

Time Duration

Most group psychotherapists conduct group sessions once a week, each session may last for 45 minutes to 1 hour.

Approaches to Group Therapy

1. The therapist role is primarily that of a facilitator he should provide a safe, comfortable atmosphere for self-disclosure.
2. Focus on the 'here and now'.
3. Use any transference situations to develop insight into their problems.
4. Protect member from verbal abuse or from scapegoating.
5. Whenever appropriate provide positive reinforcement this gives ego support and encourages future growth.
6. Handle circumstantial patients, hallucinating and delusional patients in a manner that protects the self-esteem of the individual and also set limits on the behavior so as to protect other group members.
7. Develop ability to recognize when a group member is fragile. He should be approached in a gentle, supportive and nonthreatening manner.
8. Use insight effectly to encourage introspection and facilitate insight.
9. Laughter and a moderate amount of jocking can act as a safety value and at times can contribute to group cohesiveness.
10. Role playing may help a member develop insight into the way in which he relates to others.

Steps of Group Therapy

The steps of group therapy can differ from an individual group therapist to therapist.

1. **Selecting group members**: It is very important function of a group therapist. It is based on problems of the patients.
2. **Developing contact**:
   a. The purpose should be made clean to all members in a group.
   b. Time, length, and place of the meeting should be announced.
   c. Starting and ending time and how frequently sessions will be conducted.

   d. Attendance of members.
   e. Confidentiality to be maintained.
   f. Role of the members are to respect punctuality, maintain confidentiality and interact freely.
3. **Selection of group leaders**: Role of the therapist acts as facilitator and helper.

Therapeutic Factors Involved in Group Therapy

These involve sharing experiencing, support to and from group members, socialization, imitation, and interpersonal learning.

Sharing experiences: This helps the patient to realize that they are not isolated and that other also have similar experiences and problems. Hearing from other patients that they have shared experiences is often more convincing and helpful than reassurance from the therapist.

Support to and from group members: Receiving help from other group members can be supportive to the person helped. The sharing action of being mutually supportive is an aspect of group cohesiveness that can provide a sense of belonging for patient who feel isolated in their everyday life.

Socialization: It is an acquisition of social skills (e.g. maintaining eye contact) within a group through comment that member provide about one another's deficiencies in social skills. This process can be helped by trying out new ways of interacting within the safety of the group.

Imitation: It is the learning from observing and adopting the behaviors of other group members. If the group runs well, patients imitate the adaptive behavior of the group members.

Interpersonal learning: It refers to learning about difficulties in the relationships by examining the interaction of individuals with the other member of the group.

Some Useful Techniques in the Group Therapy

- Reflecting and rewarding comments of the group members
- Asking for group reaction to member's statements
- Asking for individual reaction to one member's statements
- Point out any shared feelings within the group summarizing various points at session's end.

Advantages of Group Therapy

1. It provide opportunity for immediate feedback from a peers.
2. To observe the patient's psychological and behaviorable responses.

Role of Nurse in Group Therapy

1. To provide information to the group.

2. Selecting members according to the purpose of the group.
3. Arrange time, frequency and place for a group meeting.
4. Establishing group rules.
5. Negotiating contract with group members.
6. Share member's perception.
7. Maintain confidentiality.
8. Help the patient to know what is reality.
9. Make observation of all the nonverbal techniques being used by the patient.
10. Intervene the group by means of communication.
11. Set limits for patients.
12. Help to improve communication skills.
13. Share feelings of fear, loneliness and frustration.
14. Keep record of written notes of group sessions.

CONCLUSION

Group therapy gives an opportunity for immediate feedback from a patient's peer and a chance for both the patient and therapist to observe the patient's psychological, emotional and behavioral response toward a variety of peoples. Thus it helps the patient to master communication and interpersonal skills, problem-solving, decision-making, assertiveness skills thus enabling him to recenter the society's mainstream with a greater degree of confidence.

SUPPORTIVE THERAPY

Introduction

It is a form of 'surface therapy'. The therapist helps the client to relieve emotional relieve, emotional distress and symptoms without probing into the part or attempting to change or alter the basic personality of the individual.

Definition

According to Lawrence Rockland (1989) described 'supportive therapy'. It is widely used in hospitals and in the community settings; utilizes many psychodynamic theories whereby people will understand how to adopt, e.g. birth, childhood, puberty, marriage, death, etc. everything is considered as family experiences. Family is a source of emotional attachments.

'It is a form of psychological treatment given to patient with chronic and disabling psychiatric condition for whom basic charge is not seen as a realistic goal'.

Goals

- Support reality testing

- Provide ego support
- Maintain or re-establish usual level of functions.

Selection Criteria

1. Very healthy individual faced with overwhelming crises.
2. Patient with ego deficits.
3. Patient with alexithymia or passiveness (those with a striking inability to find words to describe once emotions and a tendency to describe endless situation details or symptoms instead of feelings).

Duration

Days, months or years are needed.

Techniques of Supportive Psychotherapy

- Ventilation
- Reassurance
- Environmental modification
- Guidance and suggestions
- Persuasion
- Explanation
- Re-education.

1. **Ventilation**—It is a free expressions of feelings or emotions. The patient is allowed to talk freely whatever comes to his mind. The client is encouraged to talk about problems. It helps the client to unburden his feelings by sharing and revealing, e.g. a student feels that her way of talking to the teacher was not appropriate. She feels it and becomes uncomfortable or tense until a day she gets an opportunity to talk to the teacher and ask for apology. The teacher might not have been thought of the harshness in the student's behavior.
2. **Environmental modification or manipulation**—A method of improving the well-being of mental patients by changing their living conditions, if there is a restless patient in the ward due to other patient may be transferred to a cubicle where no other patient allowed for a day or two.
3. **Persuasion**—It is used in which the therapist attempts to induce the patient to modify his faulty behavior by using his power of reasoning, will and slef-criticism, e.g. a mother who is neglecting her girl-child may be helped to modify her behavior.
4. **Re-education**—The patient's learns more effective way of dealing with problems and relationship through therapist-patient relationship or group therapy.
5. **Reassurance**—It is a supportive approach that encourages the patient to believe that there are possibilites of improvement, it is

also used to diminish anxiety, e.g. by explaining to the patient that the period of heightened depression is a temporary phase.

6. **Explanation**—The therapist encourage the provision of explanations of such diverse matters as the nature of the patient's symptoms, choice of treatment and likely outcomes.
7. **Guidance and suggestions**—It involves the provision of direct and indirect advice to handle the problems, e.g. job interview, contact with other members.

Principles

- Patient therapist relationship has to be established.
- The setting for supportive therapy has to allow for activity.
- This therapy will be used as adjunct to other therapies.
- Involvement of the family and social support system.
- It focuses on present problems of the patient and immediate help has to be provided.
- Supportive measures and problem-solving approaches in the therapeutic sessions has to be provided like advice, education, limit setting, environmental manipulation, and counseling.

Indications

- Schizophrenia
- Borderline personality disorders
- Anxiety
- Posttraumatic stress
- Eating disorders
- Substance abuse
- Psychosis
- Crisis.

Role of the Therapist

- The therapist has to possess specific qualities like empathy, concern, nonjudgemental, acceptance,willingness, genuine interest, and respect.
- Therapist will play an active role, directive, and supportive role. He helps the client to improve social functioning and coping skills.
- Therapist will promote two way communication process by encouraging the client to talk more about his life events.
- Motivates the client autonomy to adopt treatment modality and life decisions.
- Identifies the patient's strength, abilities, and coping skills.
- Help them to utilize biopsychosocial coping resources to achieve independent living skills.
- Tries to reduce the client's subjective feelings, distress, and maladaptive coping responses.

Chapter 11 Family Therapy

INTRODUCTION

It is a form of group psychotherapy in which the family is a therapeutic unit. Family is the matrix out of which all human interactions develop. The objective of the family therapy is not merely to improve the relationship but to modify home influences that contribute to the disorder of one or more family members.

In this therapy the therapist also encourages the member to communicate more meaningfully and handle their difficulties in a constructive manner.

Family is the most powerfull primary social system or primary social group, to which a person ever belongs. For example, birth, childhood, puberty, marriage, death, etc. everything is considered as family experiences. Family is a source of emotional attachments where an individual experiences all type of emotion whether it is positive or negative within the family. Every individual within the family has certain roles and responsibilities. The overriding value in family's lies in the relationships is essential to provide the primary context of human development.

Most family therapist identifies the individual psychiatrist problems which are inseparably related to the family in which he lives. Thus the focus of the therapy is not an individual client alone, the family or the situational support also take into consideration.

OVERVIEW OF FAMILY THERAPY

Family therapy is broadly defined as 'the attempt to modify the relationship in a family to achieve harmony.' A basic assumption of the family therapy is that there are certain human behavior pattern that can help people grow and live creatively, while there are others that lead to dysfunction and noncommunicative action and result in emotional illness in the family.

In family therapy, family is viewed as a system in which members are interdependent, a change in one part (member) of the system affects or create change in all the parts. The focus is not an individual identified client but rather on the family as a whole. The basic concept of this form of treatment is that, it is more logical faster, more satisfactory and more economical to treat all members of a system of relationships than to concentrate on the person who is supposed to be in need of treatment.

Definition

A psychotherapeutic approach that focuses on altering interactions between a couple within nuclear family and other personal systems with the goal of alleviating problems initially presented by individual family members, family subsystems, the family as a whole or other referral sources.

Aims

- Changes the relationships through changing the interactions among the people who makeup the family or marital unit.
- Family therapist evaluates the complexes web of relationships, pattern of transaction that repeats themselves and unspoken rules that derives the transactions.
- Improves group interactions and help each member to function efficiently.
- Reduce the dysfunctional behavior and interaction of individual family member.
- Reduce interfamily relationship conflicts.
- Mobilize family resources in problem solution.
- Encourage adaptive family problem-solving or coping behavior.
- Improve family communication skills.
- Meet the emotional needs of the family members.
- Strengthen the family ability to cope up with major life stressors.
- Improve the integration of family system into the social system.
- Accept the illness of family members.
- Understand treatment regimen and extends their cooperation in implementation of treatment and follow-up services.
- Assist to locate the community resources.
- Reduce family stress and anxiety and establishes balance in the family life.

Indications

- Relational problem within the family unit
- Psychoses
- Schizophrenia
- Reactive depression
- Anxiety disorders
- Psychosomatic disorders
- Uncontrolled anxiety
- Hostility
- Substance abuse
- Childhood disorders
- Bipolar disorders.

Components

Assessment

- Family structure
- Role/responsibilities and functions
- Boundaries and limitations
- Communication pattern and skills
- Resources
- Problem-solving skills.

Teaching

- Communication skills.
- Problem-solving skills.

Writing behavioral and marital contract.
Assignments, e.g. homework, and problem-solving situations.

Client Selection

Families may be referred by—

- Private physician
- Welfare agencies, e.g. school, parole officers, and judges
- Family physician
- Emergency room psychiatric OPD, e.g. after crises within the family and drug abuse.
- After discharging from psychiatric hospital for follow-up services.
- Marital and sibling conflicts.
- Situational crisis and maturational crises, e.g. birth of a child and sudden death of family member.

Function of Family

Family counselors evaluate the areas of family functions or the activities which are associated with family life. Healthy families will guide the individuals, how they function in intimate relationships in the workplace, within their culture and in the society in general.

Management

Use of decision-making power for all activities, rule making, provision of financial and other support, successful negotiations with extrafamilial systems with present and future planning.

Boundary function

Boundaries will maintain a distinction between individuals within the family. Clear boundaries define the roles of members within the family and allow for differences among members. Diffused boundaries are blending together the roles, thought, and feeling of the individual; rigid boundaries prevent family members from trying out new ideas.

Communication function

Communication pattern are vital in the family life, healthy communication within the family encourages its members to express their feelings and emotions appropriately. Open expression of feelings is always essential; whatever it may either joy or sorrow or conflicts or angry; healthy communication will always help the family members to solve their problems.

Supportive function

Healthy families are concerned with each other needs, most of the time physical and emotional needs are met, they feel support from those around and are free to grow and explore new roles and fact of their personalities.

Socialization function

Socialization skills are learnt by each individual within the family. They learn how to interact negotiate and plan, adopts coping skills. Child learns how to function effectively within their family and they apply skills in their societies. Parents are primary socializing agents, where the child learns the pattern of socialization within their families. Each phase of individual life will bring new demands and require new approaches to deal with the changes. Healthy family use flexibility to adapt to the new roles.

Biological function

Replacement of species through the propagation of progeny. Family is a medium where the sex relations are controlled and regulated.

Psychological function

Love, belongingness, affection, intimate relationship, sympathy, attention, emotional stratification, care of offsprings, sexual relationship, companionship, intimacy, etc. will be attained through family.

Educational function

Mother is the first teacher and primary caregiver, who will take care of children. Child's personality and character formation will be attained through family; it exercises more influence on the body and mind of the child where his personality will be moulded.

Protective function

Protect the interest of the child, provide security to cultivate healthy behavior.

Recreational function

Family create an atmosphere where the child's interest can be fulfilled, the family provide attainment for all its members. The love among family members will create positive interest in the child.

Religious function

Family develops religious thoughts, kind heartedness and fellow belonging. The child learns moral values, ethics codes, honesty truthfulness, traditions and religious patterns through family.

Cultural function

Family moulds its members according to its culture; family serves as an instrument for transmission and continuity of culture. It transmit ideas, folkways, mores, customs, traditions, belief and values from one generation to another generation.

Social function

- Maintain social status and control member's activities.
- Accumulates and transmits social heritage and contact with all its members.
- Provide physical shelter, food, clothing which are necessary to the existence of life.
- It is a primary socializing agency and basic institutions.
- Every member within the family will try to maintain total family health status.
- Promotes safety and security and lays emphasis on kinship patterns.
- Elders in the family will teach the behavior of each individual in an accepted manner and work for effective performance of the individual within society.

APPROACHES TO FAMILY THERAPY

The family therapy come into existence between 1960 and 1970s, when therapist observed the effects of social milieu on their clients and interpersonal model is more effective.

Double-blind Theory

It describes a situation in which two conflicting messages are given simultaneously on two levels, verbal and nonverbal. As the message is conflict people find themselves in a double-blind, in which no acceptable response exists.

Strategic Model

By changing any single element in the family system, change can be brought about in the entire system. This model aim to change the patterns, the rules and the meaning of family interactions.

Family therapist will work with the family to change their rigid pattern of communication, allowing children to be present when important decisions are being made. This intervention results in a systematic change in the family communication.

Structural Model

It is based on a normative concept of a healthy family, emphasizing the boundaries between family and subsystem and the establishment, maintenance of clear hierarchy based on parental competence. The therapist would emphasize the importance of flexibility in the family system that would allow for changes inherent to normal growth and development.

Family System Theory

It decreases emotional reactivity and to encourage differentiation among individual family members.

Insight-oriented family theory

It improves insight into problematic relationships; family is an emotional system, and is responsible for its own solutions. The therapist uses nurturing and identifies dysfunctional communication pattern.

BEHAVIORAL FAMILY THERAPY

It focuses on organizational patterns, boundary systems and subsystems, it clarifies boundaries, restructures dysfunctional boundaries, changes repetitive and maladaptive interaction patterns, prescribe rituals; it changes cognitive behavior and helps in skill training. Family's specific values, norms, traditions, roles and rules have to be conceptualized, family emotional system are verified, intergenerational system, various system are passed down through the generations. The messages and legacies of the multigenerational family relate in some way to the client's presenting problem. Construct multigenerational issues by constructing a genogram. Family therapist will analyze the genogram patterns and advice the suggestions accordingly.

TYPES OF FAMILY THERAPY

Each family member will have single family therapist; they will workout on specific issues that have been defined by individual members; occasionally the family members will meet along with their therapist to observe how each member will be relating to one another in solving the issues.

Single Family Therapy

Family interaction is the focus of therapy. Family therapist observe the family interaction patterns helps the family members to clearly define the problem which were pointed out by the family member and suggests the way or solutions to attack the problem and help the family members to implement the activities, evaluate its effects and if needed, modified strategies will be taken. Nuclear families will be considered in single family therapies.

Couple Therapy /Marital Therapy

Whenever, there relational problems among the couple or marital unit, family therapy will be considered, couples together visit the family therapist; therapist will observe the family patterns, interaction, communication styles, each partner's goals, hopes, and expectations and suggest certain methods or way to solve the problem or to find a common ground to the resolve the conflicts. Partners have to recognize and respect each others similarities and differences. Certain time will be allotted to resolve the issue; if the problem was not solved alternative strategy will be adopted; repeated counseling sitting may be required with both the partners together to implement alternate strategies in order to solve family problem.

Multiple Family Group Therapy

This therapy encourages the family members to formulate new relationships outside the group, it provide support for all the families. It improves the interaction pattern, social skills, individual responsibilities among the group, method of confronting and dealing with common problems, issues, ability to function well in home and within the community.

In this therapy 4–5 families meet weekly to discuss about their problems and dealing the issues which are common to them. For example meeting within the apartments, families who have hospitalized a member in an inpatient setting.

Multiple Impact Therapy

It is more intense and time limited, focuses on developing social skills and working together as a family and with other families within the community.

Several families will live together and deal with pertinent issues related to each family member in context of the group. Several therapists come together with the families in community settings.

Network Therapy

It includes 40–60 like family members, friends, neighbors, well-wishers, professional groups, who invested in the outcome of the current crises. Thus therapy may be conducted within the family or in community itself. A person or group of individuals invested efforts and resources, now they are experience certain crises. The groups know each other and interact on a regular basis.

In the network therapy people will mobilize their energy with efforts; definitely the reward will be more and effective. Therapist will guide the group members by clarifying the issues, reinforces the importance; emphasizes on collective effort, assist in development and effective management in problem solution.

Psychoeducational Family Therapy

It will be effective, especially as a family treatment modality combined with other modalities like psychopharmacology.

Indications

- Cases of schizophrenia
- Medical cases.

Aims

- Family works promotes and supports families in coping with a family member with severe mental illness.
- Sharing of mental health care information.
- It helps family members to understand better about their family member's illness, prodromal symptoms, medications needed to reduce symptoms, strategies in dealing with problems.
- Feelings of stigmatization, sadness, helplessness and hopelessness, etc. can be shared.
- It may be helped in parent management training, e.g. working with conduct disorder child.

CHARACTERISTICS OF DYSFUNCTIONAL FAMILIES

Families who experience emotional difficulties usually have communication problems. They may discount or ignore each other's communication.

They may 'scapegoat' on of their members by viewing and treating that member as though he or she is the cause of all the family's problems. They may create 'triangles' in which two family members from an alliance and exclude the third person. Passive-aggressive behavior is common.

FAMILY-CENTERED APPROACH

Family therapy is therapy for the entire family. It is based on the beliefs that the behaviors of one person in the family affects everyone in the family, and that the presence of symptoms such as depression or anger in one family member is a sign of disorder, pain or problem in the whole family systems. The behavior of an individual cannot be understood without understanding the behavior of other family members. Interventions are directed as the family as a whole and their behaviors, not at an identified client. Family therapy promotes family cohesion.

TECHNOLOGY FOR FAMILY THERAPY

Genogram— A three generational map of family structure and relationships which may be used to diagnose and understand family's history, problems, roles and values.

Communication technique include—

- Discussing painful events or family problems openly.
- Clarifying members thoughts, feelings and messages.
- Dealing with anger openly and nonjudgmental.
- Connecting feelings and facts, never blaming.
- Expressing empathy with family members.
- Experimental and homework activities, such as planning a family vacation, doing a fun activity together or eating meals together.
- This therapy will be used as adjunct to other therapies.
- Involvement of the family and social support system.
- If focuses on present problems of the patient and immediate help has to be provided.
- Supportive measures and problem-solving approaches in the therapeutic sessions has to be provided like advice, education, limit, setting environmental manipulation, and counseling.

APPLICATION OF NURSING PROCESS IN FAMILY THERAPY

Assessment

Assessment of family system, subsystem and individual within the family is required. A careful analysis of sound assessment will help the team members to identify the appropriate family intervention for solution of family problem.

Essential information has to be gathered related to—

- Sociocultural issues

- Past medical and mental illness
- Family interaction
- Communication pattern
- Area of stress within the family
- Pattern of family life cycle
- Multigenerational issues
- Developmental crises
- The skill related to parenting, problem-solving
- Conflict management
- Limit setting.

Nursing Diagnosis

The problems related to relational problems, abuse or neglect or bereavement has to be identified, e.g.

- Impaired adjustment
- Impaired parenting
- Sexual dysfunction
- Interrupted or dysfunctional family processes
- Strain for caregiver
- Spiritual distress
- Defect in utilization of defense/coping mechanisms
- Impaired communication pattern.

Planning

Nurse-clinician has to determine the immediate and long-term needs of family and formulate its goals, interventions. Nurse-clinician has to be nonjudgmental in presenting the information, as well as in tone of voice and responses given.

Nurse-clinician helps the family members to learn about illness, medications, situational support and availability of resources, measures for improving quality of life.

Nursing Interventions

- Nurse-clinician will provide counseling by the use of problem-solving approach to meet immediate difficulty of individual within the families.
- Advanced session motivate the families to develop and practice good listening skills, positive attitude, nonjudgmental type of practices.
- Critical observation has to be notified to make appropriate interventions in a timely manner.
- Sometimes informal conversation also will have greatest effect.
- A few general guidelines will help the nurse-clinician to be nonjudgmental in the information presented, as well as the tone of voice and question asked.

- Nurse consider the family's culture, ethnicity, socioeconomic status, families cycle, attitude toward illness which will affect individuals health and its progress and response to case management while planning and implementing nursing interventions.

Interventions are:

- Case management
- Psychoeducation
- Appropriate referrals
- Provision of emotional support and guidance and counseling
- Utilization of community resources
- Utilizes various theoretical approaches in provision of family interventions.

Evaluation

Nurse-clinician will observe whether the family is able to co-operate in provision of care to meet the client's needs within the family and in society where they are living; if they are co-operating and fulfilling their needs the frequency of family therapist visits will be reduced otherwise for implementing modified strategies the counseling sessions frequency will be increased.

Chapter 12 Behavior Therapy

INTRODUCTION

Behavior is considered to be maladaptive when it is age inappropriate, when it interferes with adaptive functioning or when others misunderstand it in terms of cultural inappropriate. The behavioral approach to therapy is that people have become what they are through learning processes or more correctly through the interaction of the environment with their genetic endowment. The basic assumption is that problematic learning and therefore can be corrected through the provision of appropriate learning experiences.

OVERVIEW

It is a form of psychotherapy which focuses on modifying faulty behavior rather than basic changes in the personality instead of probing the unconscious or exploring the patient's thoughts and feelings, behavior therapist tries to eliminate the symptoms and modify ineffective or maladaptive pattern by applying basic learning techniques.

DEFINITION

It is the systematic application of principles of learning to the analysis and treatment of disorder of behavior.

PRINCIPLES OF BEHAVIOR THERAPY

The principles of behavior therapy are based on the early studies of:
a.Classical conditioning by Pavlov (1927)
b.Operant conditioning by Skinners (1938).

Classical Conditioning

Pavlov in his experiment on dogs discovered that organisms can learn to respond in specific ways if they are conditioned to do so.

In this trials he found that the dogs salivate when they began to eat the food offered to them. This was a reflexive response called an unconditioned response. He also noticed that with time the dogs began to salivate when the food came in their range of view. Pavlov called it as conditioned response. He carried the experiment more further by presenting the food with the sound of the bell, after a number of trials with the combined stimuli (food and bell) Pavlov found that the reflexive salivation began to occur when the dog was presented with the sound of the bell in the absence of food.

Thus it was very clear that unconditioned responses (salivation) occur in response to unconditioned stimuli (eating food). He also found that a conditioned stimulus (sound of the bell) along with unconditioned stimulus could elicit the same response alone.

Sequence of conditioning operations

	Stimulus		Response
1.	UCS Unconditioned stimulus (Eating food)	⟶	UCR Unconditioned response (Salivation)
2.	UCS (Eating food)	⟶	CR (Salivation)
3.	CS Conditioned stimulus (bell)	⟶	NR No response
4.	UCS + CS (Food + bell)	⟶	CR Salivation
5.	CS (bell)	⟶	CR Salivation

Operant Conditioning

It works on the principle of law of effect, i.e. the connection between a stimulus and a response is strengthened or weakened by the consequences of the response. A stimulus that follows a behavior (or response) is called reinforcing stimulus or reinfocuses the function is called reinforcement when the reinforcing stimulus increases the probability that the behavior will recur it is called positive reinforcement. Negative reinforcement is increasing the probability that a behavior will recur by removal of an undesirable reinforcing stimulus.

Examples of reinforcing stimulus

Type	*Stimulus*	*Behavioral response*	*Reinforcing stimulus*
Positive	Messy room	Child cleans her room	Gets allowance
Negative	Messy room	Child cleans her room	Does not get scolding
Aversive	Messy room	Does not clean her room	Receives scolding from mother

Techniques for modifying client behavior

- **Shaping**: In shaping the behavior of another reinforcements are given for increasingly closer approximations to the desired response.
  For example in eliciting speech from an autistic child, the teacher must first reward the child for:
  a) Watching the teacher's lips.
  b) For making only sound in imitation of the teacher.
  c) For forming similar sounds to the word uttered by the teacher.
  It has been an effective way of modifying behavior for tasks that child has not mastered on command.
- **Modeling**: It involves learning of new behaviors by imitating the behavior in other role models are individuals who have qualities or skills that a person admires and wishes to imitate children imitate the behavior patterns of their parents, teachers and friends. In therapeutic community it can occur in a therapy session in which the clients watch a model demonstrate appropriate behavior in a role play of the client's problem. The client is instructed to imitate the models behavior in a similar role play and is positively reinforced for appropriate limitation.
- **Premack principle**: This technique named after its originator states that a frequently occurring response (R) can serve as a positive reinforcement for a response (R) that occurs less frequently. This is accomplished by allowing (R) to occur only after (R) has been performed, e.g. 13-year-old Jennie has been neglecting her homework as she spends great time on telephone talking to friends applying premack principle being allowed to talk on the telephone to her friends serve as a positive reinforcement for completing her homework.

Discriminative Stimulus (Homework to do or not to do) ⟶ R_2 (completion of homework) ⟶ R_1 (Talk to friends on home)

- **Extinction**: It is the gradual decrease in frequency or disappearance of a response when the positive reinforcement is withheld. A classic example of this technique is its use with children who have temper tantrums. The tantrum continues as long as parent gives attention to them but decrease and often disappear when the parent simply leaves the child in the room.
- **Behavior modification**: It is also called 'simple extinction' learned behavior pattern becomes a waste or disappear, if it is not reinforced. To eliminate a maladaptive behavior one has to remove the reinforcement for it. It is effective when reinforcement is being used without the knowledge of the affected individual, e.g. Rishu, 11-year-old boy, is told that if he study one hour regularly on his own in class VI he would be allowed to buy a cricket set of his own choice.

- **Contingency contracting**: In contingency contracting a contract is drawn up almost all parties involved. The behavior change that is desired is stated explicity in writing. The contract specifies the behavior charge desired and the reinforces to be given for performing the desired behaviors. The negative consequences or punishers that will be rendered for not fulfilling the terms of the contract are delineated.
- **Token economy**: Token economy is a type of contingency contracting in which the reinforces for desired behavior are presented in the form of tokens. Essential to this type of technique is the prior determination of terms and situations of significant to the client that can be employed as reinforcements, e.g. a client may be able to buy a snack, a trip to coffee shop or library or trip outside the hospital. The clients should be allowed to make the decision to whether to spend the token as soon as possible or to accumulates tokens that may be exchanged later for a more desirable reward.
- **Time out**: It is an aversive stimulus or punishment during which the client is removed from the environment where the unacceptable behavior is being exhibited. The client is usually isolated so that the reinforcement from the attention of others is absent.
- **Reciprocal inhibition**: It is also called counter conditioning reciprocal inhibition decreases or eliminates a behavior by introducing a more adaptive behavior but one that is incompatible with the unacceptable behavior, e.g. relaxation exercises are given to reduce anxiety.
- **Overt sensitization**: Overt sensitization is a type of aversion therapy that produces unpleasant consequences for undesirable behavior, e.g. disulfiram is a drug that is given for individuals who wish to stop drinking alcohol.
- **Covert sensitization**: It relies on the individuals imagination to produce unpleasant symptoms rather than on meditation. The technique is under the clients control and can be used whenever and wherever it is required. The individual learns, through mental imagery, to visualize nauseating scenes and even to induce a mild feeling of nausea. This mental image is visualized when the individual is about to succumb to an attractive but undesirable behavior. The primary advantage of covert sensitization is that the individual does not have to perform the undesired behaviors but imagines them.
- **Systematic sensitization**: This therapy was developed by J Wolpe and others. It is a technique for assisting individuals to overcome their fear of a phobic stimulus. It is systematic in that there is a hierarchy of anxiety producing events through which the individual progress diving therapy. It is based on reciprocal inhibition principle.
  a. Discuss riding an elevator with therapist.
  b. Look at the picture of an elevator.

c. Work into the lobby of a building and see the elevators.
d. Push the button for the elevator.
e. Walk into an elevator with a trusted person, disembark before the doors close.
f. Walk into the elevator with a trusted person, allow doors to close, then open the doors and walk out.
g. Ride one floor with a trusted person and then walk back down the stairs.
h. Ride one floor with a trusted person and ride the elevator back down.
i. Ride the elevator alone.

- **Steps of systematic desensitization**: The objective and 3 main steps is to reduce or eliminate fear or anxieties in which—

1. Relaxation techniques—By muscle relaxation, hypnosis, meditation, yoga, biofeedback, etc.
2. Hierarchy construction—Here the patient is asked to list all the conditions which provoke anxiety. Then he is asked to list them in a descending order of anxiety provocation.
3. Desensitization of the stimulus—This can be done by imaginary or in reality.

   – **Example**: A child is having a fear of crossing the road for a few days the mother can take the child to the road end just stand and talk about other things. The child keep observing people crossing to and fro. Then after 2 or 3 days mother and child cross the road while talking. This may reduce the anxiety in a child.

- **Indications**: Phobia
  Obsessive compulsive disorder
  Sexual disorders.
- **Flooding**: This technique sometimes called implosive therapy is also used to sensitize individuals to phobic stimuli. It differs from systematic desensitization that instead of working up a hierarchy of anxiety producing stimuli, the individual is flooded with a continuous presentation of the phobic stimulus until it no longer elicits anxiety, e.g. Intense phobia of lizard.
- **Shaping**: In shaping the components of a particular skill the behavior is reinforced step by step. The therapist starts shaping by reinforcing the existing behavior. Once it is established he reinforces the responses which are closest to the desired behavior and ignores other responses.
- **Response shaping**: Response shaping or incorporating or establishing a response which is not existing in an individual's behavior. This technique is used in behavioral problem or mental retardation, e.g. Shuban 14-year-old, has an intelligence level of 5-year-old child. He had never done any activities such as washing after defecation,

wearing shoes and shocks. The therapist trained the family member to encourage Shuban to wear his shocks and shoes. In this he can be encouraged to learn those behavior which has never learnt.

- **Chaining**: It is used when a person fails to perform a task, i.e. complex. The complex task is broken into a number of small steps and each step is taught to patient. In forward chaining one starts with the first step to second step and so on similarly in backward chaining one starts with last step and goes to the step and so on.

Operant conditioning procedures for decreasing maladaptive behavior

- **Extinction/Ignoring**: Extinction means removal of attention rewards permanently following a problem behavior. This includes action like—Not looking to the patient, not talking to the patient or having no physical contact with the patient, etc. following the problem behavior.

Operant conditioning for increasing adaptive behavior

- **Positive reinforcement**: It is a stimulus or stimulus situation which is given to the patient or individual after the response. When the stimulus is given after the response it is on the basis that strength of the response. It is on the basis that strength of the response will appear again. When a behavioral response is followed by generally rewarding event such as food, praise or gifts it tends to be strengthened and occurs more frequently than before the reward. This technique is used to increase desired behavior, e.g. as soon as the infant gets up and walks the mother claps and gives the infant a piece of chocolate to enjoy.
- **Token economy**: This program involves giving token rewards for appropriate or desired target behaviors performed by the patient. The token can later be exchanged for other rewards, e.g. on inpatient hospital wards, patients receive a reward for performing a desired behavior, such as tokens which they may use to purchase luxury items or certain privileges. It is a behavior therapy program usually conduct in a hospital or classroom setting. In token economy the desired behavior is reinforced by offering tokens that can be exchanged for special foods, games, comics and other rewards, e.g. a patient with schizophrenia does not maintain personal hygiene. The day he maintain he gets a token as reinforcer that he can watch TV when he desires, like he is able to collect may token and adapt behavior.

Operant conditioning procedures to teach new behavior

- **Modeling**: It is a method of teaching by demonstrate wherein the therapist shows how a specific behavior is to be performed. In modeling the patient observes other patients indulging in target behavior and getting reward for those behaviors. This will make the patient repeat the same behavior and earn rewards in the same manner. In which learning occur through observation. The client watches someone else perform a particular action such as—Answering the telephone. Models are often parents or other adults and children.

- **Punishment**: Aversive stimulus (punishment) is presents contingent upon the undesirable response. The punishment procedure should be administered immediately and consistently following the undesirable behavior with clear explanation.
- **Time out**: It includes removing the patient from the reward or the rewards from the patient for a particular period of time following a behavior problem, e.g. the child is not allowed to go out of the ward to play if he fails to complete the given work.
- **Restitution (over correction)**: It means restoring the disturbed situation to a state that is much better than what it was before the occurrence of the problem behavior, e.g. if a patient passes urine in the ward, he would be required to not only clean the dirty area but also mop the entire/larger area of the floor in the ward.
- **Response cost**: This procedure is used with individuals who are on token programs for teaching adaptive behavior when undesirable behavior occurs, fixed number of tokens or points are deducted from what the individual has already earned.

ASSERTIVENESS AND SOCIAL SKILL TRAINING

Assertive training is a behavior therapy technique in which the patient is given training to bring about change in emotional and other behavioral pattern by being assertive client is encouraged not to be afraid of showing an appropriate response, negative or positive to an idea or suggestion. This training is given by therapist 1st by role playing and then by practice in a real life situation. Attention is focused on more effective interpersonal skills, e.g. a timid patient will become less anxious if he is made to realize that giving voice to his feelings is appropriate such as—Complaining about poor service.

COGNITIVE THERAPY

It is a psychotherapeutic approach based on the idea that behavior is secondary to thinking our mood and feelings are influenced by our thoughts. Self-defeating and self-depreciating patterns of thinking results in depressed mood. The therapist helps the patients by correcting this distorted way of thinking feelings and behavior. This behavior therapy based on emotional problems is an individual arise due to faulty way of thinking and distorted attitude toward on self and others. The therapist takes the role of a guide who helps the patient to correct and revise his perceptions and thoughts. This helps the patient to change his thoughts, feelings and behavior about himself.

The cognitive model of depression includes cognitive triad.

1. A negative view about self
2. A negative view about the environment
3. A negative view about future.

Techniques of Cognitive Therapy

1. Teaching reattribution technique.
2. Increasing objectivity in perspectives.
3. Behavioral techniques (such as—activity scheduling homework assignments, graded task assignment).
4. Role playing and diversion techniques.
5. Teaching problem solving skills.

Indication

Cognitive therapy is used for the treatment of depression, anxiety disorder, panic disorder, phobic and eating disorders.

Schedule

A typical cognitive therapy schedule consist of about 15 visits over a 3 month period.

ABREACTION THERAPY

Abreaction is a process by which repressed material, particularly painful experience or conflict is brought back to consciousness. The person not only recalls but also relieves the material which is accompanied by the appropriate emotional response. It is most useful in acute neurotic conditions caused by extreme stress. Although abreaction is an integral part of psychoanalysis and hypnosis it can also be used independently.

Method

Abreaction can be brought about by strong encouragement to relieve the stressful events the procedure is begin with neutral topics at first and gradually approaches areas of conflict although abreaction can be done with or without the use of medication the procedure can be facilitated by giving a sedative drug intravenously. A safe method is the use of thiopentone sodium, i.e. 500 mg dissolved in 100 ml of normal saline. It is infused at a rate no faster than ice/min to prevent sleep as well as respiratory depression.

AVERSION THERAPY

Aversion therapy is used for the treatment of conditions which are pleasant but undesirable, e.g. alcohol abuse, homosexuality.

The underlying principle is the poring of the pleasant stimulus (e.g. alcohol) with an unpleasant response (e.g. brief electrical stimulus) putting a bitter taste on nails or tongue for nail biting, 20–40 session are given for 1 hours.

RELAXATION THERAPY

Relaxation produces physiological effects opposite those of anxiety slowed heart rate, increased peripheral blood flow and neuromuscular stability.

There are many methods which can be used to induce relaxation.

Jacobson's Progressive Muscular Relaxation

Patients relax major muscle groups in fixed order, beginning with the small muscle groups of the feet and working cephalad or *vice versa.*

HYPNOSIS

The word 'hypnotism' was first use by James Braid in the 19th century. Hypnosis is an artificially induced state in which the person is relaxed and unusually suggestible. Hypnosis can be induced in many ways such as by using a fixed point for attention, rhythmic monotonous instructions, etc.

Changes that Occur During Hypnosis

- The person becomes highly suggestible to the commands of the hypnotist.
- There is an ability to produce or remove symptom of perception.
- Dissociation of a part of body or emotions.
- Amnesia for the events that occurred during the hypnotic state.

Techniques

Patient is either made to lie down on a bed or sit in a chair. He is asked to gaze fixedly on a spot. Therapist makes monotonous suggestions of relaxation and sleep. The patient is however not asleep and can hear what is being said answer questions and obey instructions. This therapy is useful in:

- Abreaction of past experiences
- Psychosomatic disorders
- Conversion and dissociative disorders

- Eating disorders
- Habit disorders and anxiety disorders.

MENTAL IMAGERY

It is a relaxation method in which patients are instructed to imagine themselves in a place associated with pleasant relaxed memories. Such images allow patients to enter a relaxed state or experience a feeling of calmness or tranquility.

USE OF TAPE-RECORDED EXERCISES OR INSTRUCTIONS

It allows patients to relax on their own.

YOGA OR MEDITATION

It is concentrating on the spirit by using certain postures to prepare the body to sit motionless, remain alert and focus on one particular point, it is useful in reducing stress and anxiety.

BIOFEEDBACK

Biofeedback is based on the idea that the autonomic nervous system can come under voluntary control through operant conditioning. Thus it helps people to control usually involuntarily physiological functions so as to change them. For instance, by relaxing people learn to control these functions by hearing or seeing signals from instruments that produce information about various measures such as muscle tension, blood pressure, etc. this feedback helps the patient to control such responses.

It includes treatment of enuresis treatment of host of ailments brought on by stress such as migraine headaches, tension headaches, idiopathic hypertension, cardiac problems, etc.

CURRENT RESEARCH

Behavior therapy beyond childhood, IAN communist Thomas Frazier, PhD, the section of behavioral medicine.

Controversy and myths in autism treatment continue to proliferate throughout the parent and professional community. There are a number of myths regarding intensive behavioral treatment approaches such as applied behavior analysis (ABA).

Research on dialectical behavior therapy for patients with borderline personality disorder.

Korrner K, Linehan MM research evidence to date indicates that although DBT was developed for the treatment of patients suicidal behavior it can be adopted to treat BPD patients with comorbid substance abuse disorder and de-extended to other patient population and the treatment of other disorders.

BIBLIOGRAPHY

1. Mary TC. Psychiatric Mental Health Nursing, 5th ed. Jaypee Brothers Medical Publishers (P) Ltd. 2004; 265–9.
2. Louis SR. Basic Concepts of Psychiatric Mental Health Nursing, 7th ed. Walters Kluwer. 2001; 163–5.

Chapter 13 Hypnosis or Hypnotherapy

INTRODUCTION

It is a technique that involves varying degree of suggestibility and deep relaxation effect. The word 'hypnosis' was derived from Greek word 'hypnos' means 'sleep'. The synonyms are a 'state of dissociation', 'state of altered consciousness', 'a state of repression'. But this is a misnomer, but the hypnotized individual is not asleep rather awake alert.

Hypnotherapy is the use of hypnosis to achieve resolution of psychic-trauma and distress is used along with other form of psychotherapy.

The word 'hypnotism' was first used by 'James Braid' in the 19th century. Hypnosis is a superficial or deep trance (a somnolent state/ sleep like) resembling sleep. It is induced in a patient by suggestion of relaxation and concentrating attention on a single object. The client become highly suggestible, submissive and abandons control and response to therapist's influence. He can be induced to recall forgotten events, become insensitive to pain, gains relief from tension, anxiety and other psychological symptoms. It affects behavioral change and control of attitudes.

Hypnoanalysis or hypnotherapy is a method used to help the individual talk about feeling and conflicts about which the individual normally may not be aware of and may not talk about.

HISTORY

The phenomena of hypnosis was used by man in the earliest stage of civilization. Hypnosis has been practiced by primitive people mainly for ceremonial purposes. The sound of drums, monotonous songs and movements were used to induce a trance-like state in which the individual was highly suggestible.

JB Van Helmont said that a similar magnetic field radiates from men and it can be guided by their neils to influence directly the mind and bodies of others. FA Mensmer gave the theory of 'Animal Magnetism'.

In 1841 James Braid coined the Hypnotism and placed it on a mare national and ethical basis.

DEFINITION

1. Hypnosis is an artificially induced state in which the person is relaxed and usually suggestible. Hypnosis can be induced by many ways, such as by using a fixed point for attention, rhythmic monotonous instruction, etc.
2. Hypnosis is an altered state of intense and sensitive interpersonal relatedness between hypnotist and patient, characterized by the state of attentive, receptive, concentration with a relative suspension of peripheral awareness.
3. It is the state, where the person is able to respond to appropriate suggestion by experiencing alterations in perceptions, memory or mood.
4. It is a state of heightened focal concentration and receptivity to the suggestions of other person.
5. Hypnoanalysis refers to the method used to get the patient express his unconscious conflict under hypnosis.

OBJECTIVES

- For psychological investigation, i.e. to eilicit the nature of underlying conflicts and problems and to facilitate the recall of forgotten experiences which may be emotionally important.
- To abreact past experiences (to recall repressed memories).
- To understand the dynamics of unconscious process or behavior.
- To modify symptoms and attitudes.
- In the treatment of psychosomatic manifestations, e.g. bronchial asthma.
- To control habits like overeating, smoking.
- It is an adjunct to other form of treatment.

FACTORS

Hypnotic experience involves the following three factors:

- **Absorption**—Hypnotized individual are intensively absorbed in their trance experience.
- **Dissociation**—The intense absorption means that may routine experiences that would ordinarily be conscious occur out of ordinary conscious awareness. Such experiences can be both induced and reversed with the structural use of hypnosis.
- **Suggestibility**—While hypnotized individuals are not deprived their health, they do have a tending to accept critical instruction in trance suspending the usual conscious editing function.

MEASURING HYPNOTIZABILITY

Hypnotizability is a suitable and measurable trait. A clinical assessment of hypnotizability can become a useful starting point for the use of hypnosis in treatment.

There are many scales for many purposes, e.g.

- Stanford hypnotic susceptibility scale (SHSS) (Weitzenhoffer and Hilgard, 1959)
- Hypnotic induction profile (Spiegel, 1978).
- Stanford hypnotic clinical scale (Hilgard and Hilgard, 1975).

CLASSICAL AND OPERANT CONDITIONING THEORY (FOR HYPNOSIS)

The early influence on what has come to be social learning theory were the scientific works of John B Watson (1878–1958) and BF Skinner (1904–1990).

Using the research technique designed by Ivan Pavlov Watson showed that human learn new behavior through the process of classical conditioning. He demonstrated that the conditioned stimulus could be paired with an unconditioned stimulus to elicit a coordinated response or behavior change when the unconditioned stimulus was removed the unconditioned stimulus continued to result in the same condition response.

Skinner expanded on Watson's work stating that, learning does not only involve an association between a stimulus and response, he believes that learning occurred through association of behavior with a particular consequence. Skinner referred in this process as operant conditioning. He identifies three basic consequence and response to learning situation—Reinforcement, extinction and punishment. Reinforcement may be a positive response, which then increases a particular behavior, or it may be a negative response, also termed extinction, which remove or eliminates the behavior, punishment or an unpleasant response, reduce the frequency of behavior.

Hypnosis as Model of 'Hysteria'
Kihlstrom (1979, 1994)

• Paralysis	• Catalepsy • Challenge suggestions
• Functional anesthesias	• Analgesia • Tactile anesthesia • Blindness • Deafness
• Functional amnesia	• Posthypnotic amnesia • Posthypnotic suggestion

Indications

1. Hysteria
2. Anxiety, neurosis
3. Depression
4. Psychosomatic disorder, e.g. asthma, eczema, peptic ulcer, ulcerative colitis.

5. Tics disorder Habitual spasm and stammering.
6. Anesthesia (in patients who are apprehensive of anesthetic agents).
7. Pregnancy and labor (to induce anesthesia and for relaxation).
8. To recover lost memories.
9. Children's functional disorder, e.g. nocturnal enuresis, phobias.
10. Psychodermatological problems, e.g. warts, psoriasis, urticaria.
11. Insomnia, muteness, deafness, injury.
12. Obesity, substance abuse, eating disorders, habit control—smoking.
13. Conversion symptoms.
14. Pain syndromes, tension, neurotic habits, abnormal fears.
15. Forensic use, e.g. for the purpose of refreshing recollecting of witness and victims of crimes.

Contraindications

- Hysterical personality— The patient with hysterical character may go into so-called irreversible hypnotic state, false accusation against the hypnotist, litigation and other difficulties.
- Schizophrenia— The pseudoneurotic types of cases especially with their somatic preoccupation may be mission for anxiety or conversion disorder and may precipitate psychosis.
- Paranoid states.
- Psychotic depression.
- Obsessional state.
- Status asthmaticus.

Changes that Occur During Hypnosis Trance

1. The person becomes highly suggestible to the commands of the hypnotist.
2. There is an ability to produce or remove symptoms or perceptions.
3. Dissociation of a part of the body or emotion from the reminder may occur.
4. There is a partial or complete amnesia for the event occurring during the hypnotic trance.
5. Posthypnotic suggestions can be given just after the trance and it is followed by the hypnotized person.

   Person who are hypnotizable are in no way abnormal as compared to the rest of the population.

Techniques

1. Prepare the patient and to explain what hypnosis means, i.e. explain that it is not a state of sleep; it is not essential for amnesia to occur to obtain beneficial therapeutic results.
2. It can be explained to the patient as a state of relaxation in which his field of awareness becomes narrowed and in that state suggestion will be much more effective.

3. The patient should be seated comfortably in a chair and lying down on a couch and should be encouraged to let all muscle go loose and relaxed.
4. Ask the patient to fix at the vision on a key or a light and to give suggestion that the eyelids are getting more and more tired and will close and that the tiredness is passing over the head and down various parts of the body.
5. The confidence in the therapist and good motivation are favorable factors for hypnosis some people prefer to have the patient lying down on a couch; other prefer him to sit in comfortable chair. A variety of methods are used the common most being the use of 'fixation object' the patient is asked to gaze fixedly on a pencil or a coin or a spot on the wall or celling and the therapist make monotonous suggestion of relaxation and sleep. He tells the patient that his eyes are closing and he is getting sleepy. This suggestion goes on till the patient's eyes flicker, lower and close, and breathing takes on the characteristic of a sleeping rhythm, the patient, however, is not asleep and can hear what is being said and answer question and obey instruction.

Procedure Used

1. Suggestions and relaxation techniques.
2. Light trance—Changes in motor activity like hands feel relaxed, paresthesia are induced.
3. Medium trance—Diminished pain sensation with partial or complete amnesia.
4. Deep trance—Induced visual and auditory phenomena, deep anesthesia.
5. Posthypnotic suggestions—Where the person may be asked to perform simple tasks while under hypnosis.
6. The client in a hypnotic trance—It can recall memories that are not available in a nonhypnotic state. Some clients experience age regression, while others may describe an event in the same intensity as it occurred at that time.

PROCESS OF HYPNOTHERAPY

Hypnosis is a superficial or dup trance (a somnolent state/sleep like) resembling sleep. It is induced in a patient by suggestions of relaxation and concentrating attention on a single object. The client becomes highly suggestible, submissive and abandons control and response to therapist influence. He can be induced to recall forgotten events, become insensitive to pain, gains relief from tension, anxiety and other psychological symptoms.

Posthypnotic Effects

After the subject has been brought out of the somnambulistic state, suggestion which were giving during it can still operate and is exploited in treatment. Antebi (1963) enunciates the resistance by suggestion only in patient whose ego structure well-integrated—

- Distortion of the time concept
- Distortion of the space concept
- Link are forged in the dissociation process
- Dissociation of the personality
- Induced changes in the emotional state.
- Reinforcement of the process of concretization of the object in the patient thought process.
- Distortion of the body image.

Posthypnotic Suggestion

Some time the hypnotizer suggests to the subject that after arising from the trance he will perform a certain action, when he has directed to do something, even in complete ignorance he feel himself compelled to do that action in a semiconscious state. The influence of suggestion, after the hypnotic condition has come to an end is called 'posthypnotic suggestion' through which many kinds of symptoms of disease can be eliminated.

In the above somnambulistic state, suggestion can be which can influence the patient's mental or physical state such as easing of breathing in asthmatics. Anesthesia can be suggested and this can be localized to one limb on one eye, memories can be reactivated, regression can be induced and the patient brought back to experience again events in his earlier life which has been repressed. Hallucinatory experience may be induced. For example—

- Easing of breathing in asthmatics
- Memories can be reactivated
- Regression can be induced and the patient brought back to experience again events his earlier life which had been repressed
- Hallucinatory experiences may be induced.

Mode of action

This is one of the mysteries, EEG changes in trance phase include a decrease or slow and an increase of alpha and beta waves accompanied by an amplitude and decrease in amplitude. Variability in best hypnotic subject (the changes have also been reported during other behavioral techniques such as yoga, Zen medication and autogenic training suggesting hypnosis has something in common with these state.

Ending Hypnotic Trance

The trance period can be ended simply as hypnotizer tells the patient that at a certain signal he will get up from sleep, e.g. encounting upto number five, until the specific time is reached the patient should be awake.

When the hypnotizer has been successes in hypnotizing the subject successfully uses it many times, and can repeat it very easily in a short time again.

Objections to Hypnosis

- Hypnosis remains on the external level, it does not penetrate deep enough to remove inner tension.
- Uncooperative patients (some clients neither want to be nor can easily be hypnotized).

Precautions to be Followed in Hypnosis

1. Hypnosis should be used with sound clinical judgment in a goal directed settings.
2. The clinician should be adequately trained in reconstructive psychotherapeutic techniques and psychodynamics of interventions to avoid errors in critical judging, e.g. when a therapist commits an error while the patient is in trance state it becomes ready access for the client to adapt to the error than critically judging.

PSYCHOTHERAPEUTIC APPLICATION OF HYPNOSIS

To solve the patient's problem, hypnosis enables the psychiatrist to focus the patient's intense concentration on certain areas. The desired information can be reached more directly through hypnosis. The patient's intensified transference and attention are more focused on the treatment situation; an atmosphere of receptivity enhances his capacity for exploration and change.

Advantages

1. The adjunctive role of hypnosis lies in its ability to reduce the time needed for treatment by cutting through the patient's resistance, thereby permitting the therapist to use transference as a therapeutic device, operative in a desirable direction.
2. Restoration of the patient's previous level of self-esteem.
3. The alleviation of stress in his environment.
4. The patient reformulation of the symbolism of his symptom into a less extreme form.
5. The provision of clinical atmosphere to reorient himself in strengthening his self-respect.

Three basic strategies to control enhancement:

1. Symptom alteration
2. Attitude alteration
3. Uncovering repressed material
   - Abreaction
   - Exploration

- **Symptom alteration**: A direct guidance which keep the patient's attention away from his symptoms and concomitantly remind him, that more resourceful and effective means are available for his use in coping with problems of adaptation, e.g. a confused, disoriented person can be reestablish time, place, self-identity.
- **Attitude alteration**: The patient with an alternative attitude toward a chronic, recurrent disability or a pending problematic event and by invoking the power of compliance, patient's adaptation efficiency increased, e.g. labor pains can be endured when a mother wants to experience the birth process and to deliver her baby without chemical anesthesia.
- **Uncovering repressed material**:
  - *Simple abreaction*: The release of repressed material, e.g. this method can be employed in the patient's whose syndrome developed as a result of recent situational catastrophic experiences like war, fire accidents, of not uncovered, may develop, into traumatic neurosis.
  - *Explorative uncovering*: It means use of the hyperamnesia, i.e. possible in this state of aroused concentration and it is a valuable data collecting procedure, especially when amnesia for specific events.

Limitations

- Neurotic conflicts
- Psychotic illness
- Personality disorders.

ROLE OF THERAPIST IN HYPNOSIS

1. Maintain the good therapeutic record.
2. Provide calm and undistributable environment to the client.
3. Give proper and comfortable position.
4. Therapist use proper technique so the person becomes highly suggestible to the commands of the hypnotist.
5. Therapist should have ability to produce or remove symptoms or perceptions.
6. Therapist should have ability to dissociation of a part of body or emotions.
7. Therapist uses the tape recorder to record the instruction which allows patient to practice realization in their own.
8. Therapist use monotonous sound for the suggestion of realization and sleep.

CONCLUSION

Hypnosis is a state of artificial induced (by self or others) increased suggestibility. There is a constriction in the peripheral awareness with increased focal concentration on task at hand.

Not everyone can be hypnotized the capacity for hypnosis is called hypnotizability which can be measured in a person by using tests like eye roll sign or hand levitation test. Basically these tests measure suggestibility.

About 60% of the general population can be hypnotized but only 5%–10% reach deep hypnotic trance.

BIBLIOGRAPHY

1. Ahuja N. A Short Textbook of Psychiatry, 6th ed. Jaypee Brothers Medical Publishers (P) Ltd: New Delhi. 2007.
2. Kapoor B. Textbook of Psychiatric Nursing, 1st ed. Kumar Publishing House: New Delhi, Vol-II; 1994.
3. Neeraja KP. Essentials of Mental Health and Psychiatric Nursing, 1st ed. Jaypee Brothers Medical Publishers (P) Ltd: New Delhi, Vol I; 2006.
4. Sreevani R. A Guide to Mental Health and Psychiatric Nursing, 1st ed. Jaypee Brothers Medical Publishers (P) Ltd: New Delhi, 2006.

Chapter 14 Narcoanalysis

INTRODUCTION

Narcoanalysis is one of the individual psychotherapy. The physiological intervention used to effect the behavioral change is narcoanalysis.

The term narcoanalysis is derived from the Greek word 'Narke' (meaning 'anesthesia or torpor') and is used to describe a diagnostic and psychotherapeutic technique that use psychotherapeutic drugs, particularly barbiturates, to induce a stupor in which mental elements with strong associated affects come to the surface, where they can be exploited by the therapist.

HISTORY

The term narcoanalysis was coined by Horsley. Narcoanalysis first reach the mainstream in 1922 when Robert House, a texas obstetrician use the dry Scopolamine on two prisoners. The search was effective aids to intrigation is probably as old as man's need to obtain information from an uncooperative source and as persistence as his impatience to shortcut any tortuous path. In the annals of police investigation, physical coercion has at times been substituted for painstaking and time enquiry in the belief that direct method to produce quick results. Narcoanalysis is also known as 'narcosynthesis', 'chemical psychoanalysis' and 'psychosomatic narcoanalysis', 'truth serum', 'narcosuggestion', 'narcocatharsis', and amytal and pentothal interview.

In treating psychiatric condition 'Black Wenn' used IV sodium 'amytal injection'.

Horsley (1926) used both injection 'sodium amytal and pentothal sodium' for narcoanalysis.

DEFINITION

'It refers to the intervenous injection of drugs (sedative or stimulants) into the patient as an adjunct to psychotherapy'. It inducts sedation and the client will become more amenable to psychotherapeutic intervention.

PURPOSES

1. To facilitate the diagnosis and treatment of psychiatric illness by creating and altered state of consciousness.
2. To provide symptomatic relief for severely agitate client.
3. To ventilate the significant life experience in identifying etiological factor of mental illness.
4. To differentiate between organic disabilities from functional syndromes.

USES OF NARCOANALYSIS

Stress eating disorder, to know the information from the criminals, to know the truth, anxiety traumatic neurosis, conversion, psychosomatic disorder.

TEAM MEMBERS OF NARCOTEST

In India, the narcoanalysis test is done by a team comprising of an anesthesiologists, a psychiatrist, a clinical forensic psychologist, an audiovideographer and supportive nursing staff.

The forensic psychologist will prepare the report about the revelation, which will be accompanied by a compact disk of audiovideo recording, the strength of the revelation if necessary, is further verified by subjecting the person to polygraph and brain mapping test.

DRUGS USED IN NARCOANALYSIS

Common drug used based on client's need are:

- Sedatives, e.g. Amobarbital
- Stimulants, e.g. Methylphenidate
- Other drugs—

1. Sodium pentothal
2. Sodium amytal
3. Scopolamine
4. Truth serum.

Amobarbital

It is a drug that is a barbiturate derivative. It has sedative hypnotic and analgesic properties. It is a crystalline powder with no odor and a slightly bitter taste. Barbiturates was first manufactured in the late 19th century, these drugs depress the activity in the central nervous system and reduce activation of mental alertness.

Mode of action of barbital— The effect are produced is not certain, but some evidence suggest that barbiturates may reduce the release of excitatory neurotransmitters by neurons in many different location.

Sodium Pentothal

It is a rapid onset short-acting barbiturate general anesthetic.

Sodium Amytal

It is an immediate acting barbiturate. Sedation occur in one hour or longer and last for 10–12 hours. Sodium amytal depresses the central nervous system. It is used as a sedative for, hypnotic and anticonvulsive and for narcoanalysis. When sodium amytal is used for narcoanalysis. It may be called as 'Amytal interview'.

Scopolamine (hyoscine)

It is an anticholinergic alkaloid drug that is obtained from certain plants. Anticholinergic drugs block the impulses that passes through certain nerves. Scopolamine affects the autonomic nervous system and is used as a sedative, to prevent motion sickness, to treat eye muscle paralysis (cycloplegic), and to dilate the pupil (mydriatic).

Truth Serum

It will depress the higher cortical functions of the brain due to the lowering the higher cortical function the person enter in a hypnotic stage and he is unable to say lie on his own imagination and speak freely about their anxiety and painful memories.

Preparation of solution

Sodium pentothal is supplied as a yellowish, hygroscopic powder in a variety of different containers. Solution should be prepared aseptically with one of the three following diluents: Sterile water for injection or 9% sodium chloride injection.

Since sodium pentothal contains no added bacteriostatic agent, extreme care in preparation and handling should be exercised at all times to prevent the introduction of microbial contaminants. Solution should be freshly prepared and use promptly; when reconstituted for administration to several patients, unused portions should be discarded after 24 hours.

Complications of drugs

- Respiratory depression
- Laryngospasm
- Myocardial depression
- Extravascular infiltration
- Intra-arterial infection
- Shivering.

Management of complications of drugs

1. Respiratory depression (hypoventilation, apnea)—Pentothal should be considered to have the same potential for producing respiratory depression as an inhalation agent, and patency of the airway must be protected at all times.
2. Laryngospasm—Laryngeal and bronchial vagal reflexes can be suppressed and secretions minimize by giving atropine or scopolamine premedication and barbiturate and opiate. Use of a skeletal muscle relaxant or positive pressure oxygen will usually relieve laryngospasm. Tracheostomy may be indicated in difficult cases.
3. Myocardial depression—Arrhythmias may appear if PCO_2 is elevated, but they are uncommon with adequate ventilation and dilatation is necessary management of myocardial depression is the same as for overdose.
4. Extravascular infiltration—Extravascular injection may cause chemical irritation of the tissue varying from the slide tenderness to venospasm, extensive narcosis and sloughing. If the extravasation occur the local irritant effects can be reduced by injection of 1% procaine locally to relieve the pain and enhance vasodialation with the local application of heat which help to increase local circulation and removal of infiltration.
5. Intra-arterial Injection—The area for intravenous injection of the drug should be palpated for detection of an underlying pulsating vessels. Accidental intra-arterial injection can cause arteriospasm and severe pain. There will be reduced by the following suggestions—
   - Dilute the injected pentothal by removing the tourniquet and any restrictive garments.
   - Inject the artery with a dilute solution of papaverine, 40–80 mg or 10 ml 1% procaine to inhibit smooth muscle spasm.
   - Unless other contraindicated, institute immediate heparinization to prevent thrombus formation.
   - Consider local infiltration of an alpha-adrenergic blocking agent such as–pentolamine into the vasospastic area.
6. Shivering—After pentothal anesthesia, manifested by twitching face muscle and occasional progression to tremors of the arms, head, shoulder and the body, is a thermal reaction due to increased sensitivity of cold. The treatment consist of warming the patient with blankets, maintaining room temperature near 22°C and administered chlorpromazine.

NARCOANALYSIS TEST

The narcoanalysis test is conducted by mixing 3 gm of sodium pentothal or amytal dissolved in 3000 ml of distilled water. Narco test refers to the practice of administering barbiturates or certain other chemical substances. Most often pentothal sodium, to a subject inhibitions, in that the subject will make freely share information and feelings. A person is able to lie by using his imagination. In the narcoanalysis test, the subject inhibition are lowered by interfering with his nervous system at the molecular level. In such sleep like state effort are made to obtain probable truth about the crime.

Expert injects a subject with hypnotic like sodium pentothal or sodium amytal under the controlled circumstances of the laboratory. The dose is depend on the person's size, age, health and physical condition, the subject which is put in state of hypnotism is not in a position to speak upon his own but can answer specific but simple questions after giving some suggestions. The answers are believed to be spontaneous and semiconscious person is unable to manipulate the answer. Wrong dose can send the subject into coma or death.

Effect of Administration of Drug

The role of administration is controlled to derive the accused shrewdly into a hypnotic trance the effect of the biomolecules on the bioactivity of an individual is evident as they depresses the central nervous system, lower blood pressure, slow the heart rate. Putting the subject into a hypnotic trance resulting in luck of inhibition, the subject is then interrogated by the investigation agencies in the presence of doctors (Fig. 14.1).

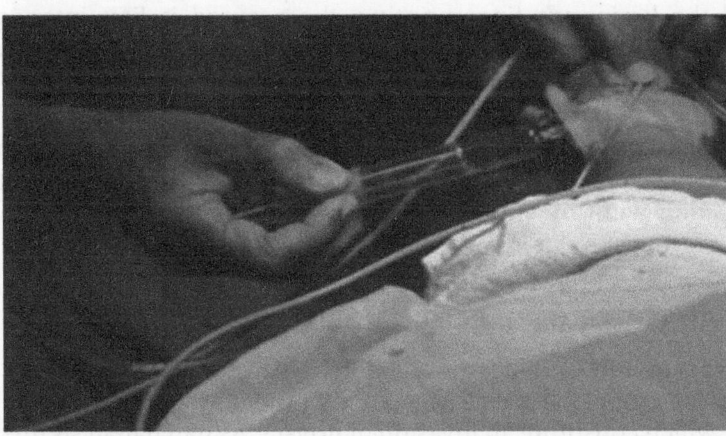

Figure 14.1: Administration of drug in narcoanalysis test

Preparation of Report

The revelation made during this stage are recorded both in video and audio cassettes, the report by the experts as what is used in the process of collecting evidence.

This procedure is conducted in government hospitals after a court order is passed instructing the doctor or hospital authorities to conduct the test personal consent of the subject is also required.

Other Associated Truth Finding Test

Apart from the narco test there are also other two kinds of tests which are popularly used on convict for extraction of truth, these are—

1. Polygraph or lie detection test
2. P300 or the brain mapping test.

Polygraph or lie detection test

It is an examination which is based on an assumption that there is an interaction between the mind and the body and is conducted by various components or the sensuous of the polygraph machine, which are attach to the body of the person who is interrogated by the experts, the machine recorded the blood pressure, pulse rate and respiration and muscle movements. Polygraph test is conducted in three phases—A pretest interview, chart recording and diagnosis. It was Keeler who further refined the polygraph machine by adding a psychogalvanometer to record the electrical resistance of the skin.

P300 or the brain mapping test

This test was developed and patented in 1995 by neurologist Dr Lawrence A Farewell, director of chief scientist. Brain wave science in this method, called the brainwave fingerprinting, the accused is first interviewed and interrogated to find out whether he concealing any information, then sensors are attached to the subject head and the person is seated before the computer monitor, he is then shown certain image or made to hear certain sound, the sensor monitor electrical activity in the brain and the register P300 waves which are generated only if the subject has connection with the stimulus, i.e. picture or same, the subject is not asked any question here.

LEGAL ASPECT OF NARCOANALYSIS

- **Right to life and personal liberty**: Narcoanalysis arguably falls within the scope of article 21 by virtue of the invasion of the body and mind, which constitute an invasion of privacy. As narcoanalysis involves the involuntary injection of mind altering drug into one's body there necessarily arises a question of whether this may constitute torture. Doctors cannot be a party of the infliction of mental or physical trauma nor aid or abet torture as per the code of ethics.
- **Impact on the right against self-indiscrimination**: Article 20(3) of the Indian constitution state that person accused of an offence shall be compelled to be a witness against himself it operates as a protection against testimonials compulsion. The Indian criminal procedure code provide that a person is seemed to truly answer all questions while being examined by the police except those that would have a tendency to expose him to a criminal penalty. The protection against self-indiscrimination is

available to both accused person who have not been charged with the commission of an offence.

- **Judicial sanction**: While the court in India have dispensed with the retirement of consent of the subject, they have also declined from exercising judicial oversight over the conduct of the test. Kerala High Court held that narcoanalysis does not require judicial sanction because it is a recognized test for an effective investigation.

The narcoanalysis test has been criticized for its unreliability scientific studies demonstrate that the test is not foolproof and even induces confession from innocent person.

Indications

- Severely agitated clients
- Hysterical amnesia
- Suicide cases
- Paranoid illness
- Organic brain syndrome
- To identify the mental symptoms such as confabulation, disorientation and denial of illness
- Schizophrenia
- Depression(stuporous depressive state)
- Legal investigation (pentothal interview).

Contraindications

- Severely cardiac impairment
- Porphyria
- Kidney dysfunction
- Liver pathology
- General disability
- Marked imaciation
- Severe anemia.

Techniques

- **Simple catharsis**—The distributing conflict is elicited with affect (abreaction, e.g. pentothal interview).
- **Suggestion**—The therapist make suggestions to the patient, while he is under the influence of the drug without attempting to uncover repressed material. It is short of supportive psychotherapy.
- **Narcoanalysis and Narcosynthesis**—Both procedures involve the subsequent application of psychotherapeutic technique to help the patient integrate and work through the material that has been elicited through the use of the drug.

Procedure

The psychiatrist has to establish a positive rapport and relationship with the patient; by establishes the relationship by altering his views of the world and his environment.

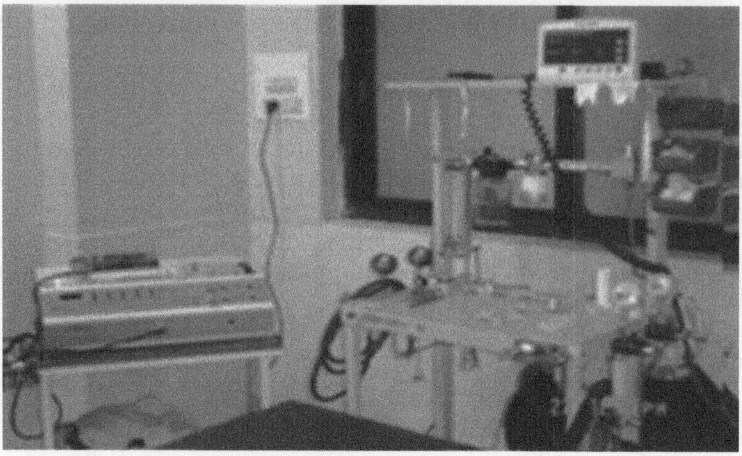

Figure 14.2: Narcoanalysis test unit

The drug will help him to relax and feel more at ease, it will permit him to talk more freely and comfortably about the feelings and experiences that bother him (Fig. 14.2).

Administration

- The drug serves a protection against the breakthrough of the anxiety which surrounds his underlying conflicts.
- The client can better tolerate expression of painful psychic material, facilities the process of exploration.
- The drug produces euphoria and weaken the inhibiting mechanisms.
- It enables the patient to tolerate painful insights and to incorporates them into his emotional and intellectual life.
- Drug should be administered in a quite room with the patient in a reclining position. (Intravenous) through antecubital vein 5% pentothal sodium in 2 minutes, at the outset the drug increases agitation or anxiety.
- Until the physician become familiar with the patient characteristic response to the drug, ask the client to count the backward from 100 immediately after the injection.
- The client falls asleep at this point, the psychological interaction between patient and therapist occurs.
- Attempt are made to discuss significant material to elicit repressed experimental date or to make appropriate suggestion.
- The patient is then permitted to go to sleep.

Postprocedural Care

- Accompany the client upto treatment room
- Rest has to be provided after the interview
- Milder dose ambulation can be allowed.

SOME NOTABLE EVENTS AND CASES OF NARCOANALYSIS IN INDIA

1. In a 2006 judgment (Dinesh Dalmia V), the Madras High Court held that subjecting an accused to narcoanalysis is not tantamount to testimony by compulsion. The court said about the accused; he may be taken to the laboratory for such test against his will, but the revelation during such test is quite voluntary.
2. In 2004, the Bombay High Court ruled in the multicrore rupee fake stamppaper case that subjecting an accused to certain tests like narcoanalysis does not violate the fundamental right against self-indiscrimination. Article 20(3) of the constitution guarantees this. No person accused of any offence shall be compelled to be witness against himself. Statements made under narcoanalysis are not admissible in evidence.
3. In January 24th 2008, a bench of chief justice KG Balakrishnan reversed its ruling after hearing arguments for three days from various parties, including solicitor general Goolam E Vahanvati and senior advocate Dushyant Dave, appointed by the Bench.

ROLE OF NURSE IN NARCOANALYSIS

1. The nurse should have several unique skills to client care, they include a perspective influences by medical model, which demands the development of hypothesis (diagnosis) tested through treatment these treatments are expected to level to specific result or changes.
2. Nurses should be knowledgeable and administrator of psychopharmacology remedies have become to prime importance.
3. The work in close partnership with psychiatrist often as key worker for client which means that they are the point of contact for client. Clients are responsible for ensuring that care planned for them actually delivered.
4. Psychonurses are trained to assess the client mental status and able to correlate the behavior or symptom shown by client and the facts which told by the client during the narco-test.
5. Nurse should assess any problem of the patient after the narco-test.
6. Therapist should explore the repressed positive and negative feeling of the patient.
7. Nurse should take consent from the patient. If the patient is mentally ill, consent should be taken from the relatives.
8. Arrange all emergency trays in the patient site.
9. Nurses act as a supporter.
10. Confidentiality should be maintained.
11. Check periodically vital signs and blood pressure.

Quality of Nurse

- Good communication skills

- Be able to work within a team structure
- Possess physical and psychological assessment skills
- Secured maturity
- Professionalism
- Confidence
- Nonjudgmental attitude
- Ability to work independently (or emergency condition)
- Knowledge about the procedure
- Ability to analysis the fact.

CONCLUSION

Narcoanalysis test is the type of individual psychotherapy. In narcoanalysis drug is used to sedate the patient and explore the findings.

Narcoanalysis is one of the individual psychotherapy. The term narcoanalysis is delivered from the Greek word 'Narke' meaning 'Anesthesia or Topor' and is used to describe diagnostic and psychotherapeutic technique that use psychotherapeutic drugs, particularly barbiturates, to induce a stupor in which mental elements with strong associated affects come to the surface, where they can be exploited by the therapist.

BIBLIOGRAPHY

1. Ahuja N. A Short Textbook of Psychiatry, 6th ed. Jaypee Brothers Medical Publishers (P) Ltd: New Delhi, 2007.
2. Kapoor B. Textbook of Psychiatric Nursing, 1st ed. Kumar Publishing House, New Delhi, Vol-II: 1994.
3. Neeraja KP. Essentials of Mental Health and Psychiatric Nursing, 1st ed. Jaypee Brothers Medical Publishers (P) Ltd: New Delhi, Vol-I: 2006.
4. Sreevani R. A Guide to Mental Health and Psychiatric Nursing, 1st ed. Jaypee Brothers Medical Publishers (P) Ltd: New Delhi, 2006.

Chapter 15 Milieu Therapy

INTRODUCTION

The word milieu is French for 'middle'. The English translation of the word is surroundings or environment. In psychiatry, therapy involving the milieu or environment, may be called milieu therapy.

The goal of milieu therapy is to manipulate the environment so that all aspects of the client's hospital experience are considered therapeutic within this therapeutic community setting the client is expected to learn adaptive coping, interaction, and relationship skills that can be generalized to other aspects of his or her life.

The therapeutic milieu is an environment that is structured and maintained as an ideal, dynamic setting in which to work, with clients. This milieu includes safe physical surroundings, all the treatment team members, and other clients. It is supported by clear and consistently maintained limits and behavioral expectations.

A therapeutic setting should minimize environmental stress such as noise and confusion, and physical stress. It provides a chance for rest and nurturance of self, a time to focus on the development of strength, and an opportunity to learn to identify alternatives or solutions to problems and to learn about the psychodynamics of those problems.

A therapeutic milieu is a safe space, a nonpunitive atmosphere in which caring is a basic factor. In this environment, confrontation may be a positive therapeutic tool that can be tolerated by the client.

Nurses and treatment team members should be aware of their own roles in this environment, maintaining stability and safety, but minimizing authoritarian behavior. Clients are expected to assume responsibility for themselves within the structure of the milieu as much as possible. Feedback from other clients and the sharing of tasks or duties within the treatment program facilitate the client's growth.

PURPOSES

A therapy approach to living experience with the following purposes:

1. Correct or redefine perception of stressors
2. Correct maladaptive behavior
3. Develop adaptive coping
4. Acquire interpersonal and stress-management skills

5. Manipulate the environment so that all aspects of clients' hospital experience are considered therapeutic
6. Client is expected to learn adaptive coping, interaction and relationship skills that can be generalized to other aspects of his or her life
7. Achieving client autonomy.

PRINCIPLES OF MILIEU THERAPY

- To promote a fundamental respect for individuals (both clients and staff).
- To use opportunities for communication between client and staff for maximum therapeutic benefit.
- To encourage client to cut at a level equal to their ability and to enhance their self-esteem.
- To promote socialization.
- To provide opportunities for clients to be part of unit management.
- Individuals are held responsible for own actions.
- Peer pressure is utilized to reinforce rules and regulations.
- Team approach is used.
- Group discussions and temporary seclusions are favored approaches for acting out behavior.
- The nurses, function is to act in way that consistently promote these goals.

CHARACTERISTICS OF MILIEU THERAPY

The concept of milieu therapy developed from a desire to counteract the negative, regressive effects of institutionalization reduced ability to think and act independently an adoption of institutional values and attitudes, and loss of commitments in the outside world.

Several strategies have been developed to counter these negative effects. They include:

- Distribution of power
- Open communication
- Structured interactions
- Work-related activities
- Community and family involvement in the treatment process
- Adaptation of the environment to meet developmental needs.

- **Distribution of power**: The milieu therapy approach involves 'flattening' the control hierarchy so all participants have a voice in decision making. This process may include the whole population of the treatment unit, or a governing council may take the final decisions based on input from various smaller groups of clients and staff members.
- **Open communication**: In therapy, treatment decisions are often made by the clients themselves, who therefore need information to make effective decision. It is not necessary to communicate personal information but clients and staff need to be aware of individual

treatment goals to ensure everyone is working towards the same goal. In this atmosphere, exclusive confidentiality is replaced by mutual trust, honesty and open communication.

- **Structured interactions**: KA Menninger pioneered the concept of structured interaction patterns in the form of attitude therapy. An advantage of the structured interaction approach is that all staff members approach the client in a consistent manner, acknowledging specific diagnostic areas, therapy shortening treatment time.
- **Work-related activities**: The focus of these activities is on benefits to the client rather than to the agency. Several factors contribute to effective work therapy programs.
  - First, clients need to choose the type of work they wish to perform.
  - Second, work activities should be geared toward developing skills that will be useful in actual job situation.
  - Third, a variety of activities provides the opportunities to test different areas for future job interest.
- **Community and family involvement in the treatment process**: Clients are kept in their usual environment, for example, a day treatment center, or halfway house, and continue most of their routine activities while receiving treatment. If one family member is hospitalized an attempt is made to continue family involvement. This is an effective way to improve family interaction and minimize the isolations resulting from hospitalizing one family members.
- **Adaptation of the environment to meet the developmental need**: To develop his full potential an individual must have an environment adapted to his current needs. Adapting the environment to meet these multiple needs is challenging due to the extension of milieu therapy to all age groups and the inclusion of family members with individuals of varying ages within the treatment milieu.

COMPONENTS

The various components of therapeutic milieu include:

1. Maintaining safe environment
2. The trust relationship
3. Building self-esteem
4. Limit setting.

Maintaining Safe Environment

The nursing staff should follow the policies with regarding to prevention of routine safety hazards and supplement these policies as necessary for example:

- Dispose of all needles safely and out of reach of client
- Restrict or monitor the use of matches and lighters
- Do not allow smoking
- Remove mouthwash, aftershave lotions and so forth, if substance abuse is suspected.

Listed below are the most restrictive measures to be used on a unit on which clients who are exhibiting behavior directly threatening or harmful to themselves or others may be present. These measures may be modified based on the assessment of the client's behavior:

- Immediately on the client's admission, search the client and all of the client's belongings and remove potentially dangerous items, such as wire, clothes, hangers, ropes, belts, safety pins, scissors and other sharp objects, weapons and medications; keep these belongings in a designated place inaccessible to the client.
- Be sure mirrors, if glass, are securely fastened and not easily broken.
- Keep sharp objects, e.g. scissors, pocket knives, knitting needles out of reach of clients and allow their use only with supervision; use electric shavers when possible (disposable razors are easily broken to access blades).
- Identify potential weapons, e.g. mop handles, hammers and dangerous equipment, e.g. electrical cords, scalpels and keep them out of the client's reach.
- Do not leave cleaning fluids, bleach, mops and tools, unattended in client care areas.
- Do not leave medicines unattended or unlocked.
- Keep keys to unit door, medicines on your purse at all times.
- Be aware of items that are harmful if ingested, e.g. mercury in manometers, thermometers.
- Search package brought in by visitors, explain the reason for such rules briefly, and do not make any exceptions.

The Trust Relationship

One of the keys to a therapeutic environment is the establishment of trust. Both the client and the nurse must trust that treatment is desirable and productive. Trust is the foundation of the therapeutic relationship, and limit setting and consistency are its building blocks.

Building Self-esteem

Strategies to help build or enhance self-esteem must be individualized and built on honesty and on the client's strengths. Some general suggestions are:

- Set and maintain limits.
- Accept the client as a person.
- Be nonjudgmental at all times.
- Structure the client's time and activities.
- Have realistic expectations of the client and make them clear to the client.
- Initially provide the client with tasks, responsibilities and activities that can be easily accomplished, advance the client to more difficult tasks as he progresses.

- Praise the client for him accomplishments however small, giving sincere appropriate feedback for meeting expectations, completing tasks, fulfilling responsibilities, and so on.
- Never flatter the client.
- Use confrontation judiciously and in a supportive manner, use it only when the client can tolerate it.
- Allow the client to make his own decisions whenever possible. If the client is pleased with the outcome of his decision, point out that he was responsible for the decision and give positive feedback.
- If the client is not pleased with the outcome, point out that the client like everyone can make and survive mistakes, then help the problem, give positive feedback for the client's taking responsibility for problem-solving and for his efforts.

Limit setting

Setting and maintaining limits are integral to a trust relationship and to a therapeutic milieu. Before stating a limit explain the reasons for limit setting. Some basic guidelines for effectively using limit are:

- State the expectations or the limit as clearly, directly and simply as possible.
- The consequence that will follow the client's exceeding the limit also must be clearly stated at the outset.
- The consequences should immediately follow the clients' exceeding the limit and must be consistent, both over time and among staff (each staff member must enforce the limit).
- Consequences are essential to setting and maintaining limits, they are not an opportunity to be punitive to a client. In conclusion, the nurse works with other health professionals in an interdisciplinary team; the interdisciplinary teamworks within a milieu that is constructed as a therapeutic environment, with the aim of developing a holistic view of the client and providing effective treatment.

ADVANTAGES AND DISADVANTAGES OF MILIEU THERAPY

Advantages

1. Milieu therapy creates a different type of attitude and behavior in the patient because the environment is like home.
2. Instead of adopting a sick role, the patient makes, decisions in the word management and cares for other patients in other words, he becomes less dependent and passive.
3. The patient learn to adopt a behavior which is acceptable in the therapeutic environment like learns to control hostility.
4. The patient learns to make decisions which improves his self-confidence.
5. Milieu includes safe physical surroundings, all the treatment team members, and other clients, which is supported by clear and consistently maintained limits and behavioral expectations.

6. A therapeutic milieu is a safe space, a nonpunitive atmosphere, which minimize the environmental stress and provides a chance for rest and nurturance of self, a time to focus on the developments of strengths, and an opportunity to learn to identify alternatives or solutions to problems and to learn about the psychodynamics of those problems.
7. Patient develops harmonious relationships with other members of the community.
8. Develops leadership skills.
9. Becomes sociocentric.
10. Learns to live and think collectively with the members of the community.

Disadvantages

1. Role blurring between staff and patient
2. Group responsibility can easily become nobody's responsibility
3. Individuals needs and concerns may not be met
4. Patient may find the transition to community difficult
5. Milieu therapy is limited to only hospitalized patients
6. Conflict resolution is needed as part of the staff skills
7. Low client-to-staff ratio
8. Requires continuous open communication among all staff and clients.

ROLE OF A NURSE IN MILIEU THERAPY

1. A nurse participating in the design or renovation of the setting can greatly affect the therapeutic physical environment.
2. A nurse input concerning the number of activities and interactions that occurs in a dayroom can determine if the design is functional.
3. The nurse may interpret the needs of the client population for design experts with knowledge of color, texture and lighting. All these factors combine to promote perceptual clarity and orientation.
4. The nurse is often responsible for making referrals, encouraging client participation and coordinating the team members involved.
5. Intervening communication pattern effectively is the most significant role of a nurse.
6. The nurse must make sure that physical environment is structured to provide both private places for contemplation and reflection and large areas for group interaction.

RESEARCH REVIEW

1. **John G Gunderson**

Department of psychiatrists, Harvard Medical School, and Director of Psychotherapy.

Until recently almost all the controlled research on milieu therapy for schizophrenic patients involved nonintensive milieu and chronic patients. Under these circumstances the effectiveness of milieus was not evident. Recent studies have suggested that intensive milieus significantly benefit nonchronic patients. This study have indicated the importance of defining what ingredients can make a milieu therapeutic. The existing research evidence is surveyed at the nature of what some of these ingredients might be described.

[A re-evaluation of milieu therapy for nonchronic schizophrenic patients].

2. **P Vaglum, S Friis, S Karterud**

[Why are the results of milieu therapy for schizophrenic patients contradictory? An analysis based on four empirical studies].

The result of milieu therapy with psychotic patient have been highly conflicting because of unrecognized differences among the wards investigated.

Our own research indicates that for psychotic patients in short and intermediate-term wards: A beneficial milieu has a low perceived level of anger and aggression and a high level of support, practical orientation, and order and organization.

Confronting group therapy is detrimental and individually oriented milieu therapy beneficial.

Community groups may become antitherapeutic pseudogroups. Extensive use of confrontational groups may contribute to a detrimental ward atmosphere. A high mean age of patients may contribute to a favorable low level of aggression. A high percentage of psychotic patients, a high number of patients, and a high staff turnover may lead to a detrimental atmosphere.

On this basis we tried to change the milieu on a 26- bedded therapeutic community ward which proved to have pseudogroups and a detrimental ward atmosphere.

The amount of compulsory group activities was reduced, the groups made more task-oriented, the amount of individually oriented milieu therapy increased, and the number of beds reduced. At re-evaluation the ward atmosphere had improved considerably.

BIBLIOGRAPHY

1. Sreevani R. A Guide to Mental Health and Psychiartic Nursing, 2nd ed. Jaypee Brothers Medical Publishers(P) Ltd: New Delhi, 193–5.
2. Townsend MC. Psychiatric Mental Health Nursing, 5th ed. Jaypee Brothers, Medical Publishers (P) Ltd. FA Davis Company: Philadelphia, 184–90.

Chapter 16

Therapeutic Community

INTRODUCTION

Therapeutic environment means safe surrounding environment. The members of the therapeutic community is usually known as, residents, clients or members.

The concept of therapeutic community was first developed by Maxwell Jones in 1953. He wrote a book entitled 'Social Psychiatry', which was first published in England. Later on when it was published in the United States, its title was changed to ' Therapeutic Community'.

DEFINITIONS

- Stuart and Sundeen defined therapeutic community as 'a therapy in which patient's social environment would be used to provide a therapeutic experience for the patient by involving him as an active participant in his own care and the daily problems of his community.'
- 'The total resources of the staff, the residents, their relatives and the institution are pooled for the purpose of treatment'.

GOALS

- Changes maladaptive behavior into adaptive behavior.
- Provide conducive environment (free and favorable climate) in which the client can talk and be aware about his feelings, impulses and behavior.
- Minimize prolongation of hospital stay.
- Promotes early recovery.
- To make the client to understand how their behavior will be affected, with the behavior of others.
- To enable the client to actively participate in his daily living activities and will be actively involved in community activities.
- Staff members will help the client to take their own decisions to solve their problems and assist in planning and implementing the community activities to solve the problem at large. Co-operation of the administration is in the hands of residents, through staff will be in authority position.

- To improve the self-esteem by allowing the client to take their own decision and taking their opinions to solve the resident's problem.
- To promote group and social interaction, every member in the group will be aware of their roles, limitations, and responsibilities.
- The client is expected to learn adapting or coping techniques, interaction, and relationship skills that can be generalized to other aspect of his life.
- Residents will be co-obligates in the formulation of the rules and regulations for the community.
- To promote the self-confidence, independence and to have self-control over their personal activities.
- To manipulate the environment so that all aspects of the client's hospital experience are considered to be therapeutic to minimize antitherapeutic environment.
- To resocialize the client.

OBJECTIVES

- To use patient's social environment to provide a therapeutic experience for him.
- To enable the patient to be an active participant in his own care and become involved in daily activities of his community.
- To help the patient's for solving problems, plan activities and develop the necessary rules and regulations for the community.
- To increase their dependence and gain control over many of their own personal activities.
- To enable the patients become aware of how their behavior affects others.

BASIC ASSUMPTIONS OF THERAPEUTIC COMMUNITY

BF Skinner has described the basic assumptions of therapeutic community as—

- Every individual will have certain abilities, strength, limitations. The capabilities of each individual has to be recognized and utilized as a foundation for personality growth, which will help the person to function more productively and effectively to adapt himself in all aspect of their life.
- Interpersonal interactions, communication, developed skill and structured situations will provide learning opportunities for the client; every interaction facilities are an opportunity for therapeutic intervention. Immediate feedback of personal perceptions will facilitate learning among the clients.
- Clients are given freedom to take decisions, autonomy and an opportunity to fulfill the basic needs of an individual and in a group setting.
- To bring behavioral modification among the client by inculcating the feeling of responsibility for their own behavior.
- Behavioral group norms are established, peer pressure is a powerful tool, direct feedback acceptable behavior are essential.

- Make the client to understand how their behavior either appropriate or inappropriate will affect the other group members.
- Avoid restriction and punishment; group discussions are made to deal with the coping methodology for overcoming destructive behavior.

ELEMENTS OF THERAPEUTIC COMMUNITY

- Free communication
- Shared responsibilities
- Involvement in decision-making
- Understanding of roles, responsibilities, limitations, and authorities
- Manipulation of environment to fulfill their needs and demands.

COMPONENTS OF THERAPEUTIC COMMUNITY

Daily Community Meetings

- These meetings are composed of 60–90 patients. All levels of unit staff are involved; including administrative personnel. Acute patients are not involved in the meetings.
- Meeting should be held regularly for 60 minutes.
- Discussion should be focus on mainly on day to day life in the unit.
- During discussions patients feelings and behaviors are examined by other members.
- Frank discussion are encouraged, these may takes place with much out pouring of emotions and anger.

Patient Government or Ward Council

- The purpose of the patient government is to deal with practical unit detail such as house-keeping functions, activity planning, and privileges.
- A group of 5–6 patients will have specific responsibilities, such as house-keeping, physical exercise, personal hygiene, meal distribution, a group to observe suicidal patients, etc. staff members should be available always.
- All decisions should be feedback to the community meetings.

Formal Training, it Provides

- Practical working experience
- Supervised practice
- Theoretical tuition for individual, group and organizational functioning and models of therapeutic change
- Personal therapeutic experience as a resident.

Staff Meeting Review

- A staff meeting should be held following each community meeting (patients are excluded and only staff are present). In this meeting the staff would examine their own responses, expectations, and prejudices.

Living and Learning Opportunities

- Learning opportunities are to be provided within the social milieu, which should provide realistic learning experiences for the patients.

Conditions which are required for the promotion of therapeutic community.

Everything within the client's environment is considered as a part of therapeutic environment or treatment program. The community setting or the community factors like social interactions, schedule of activities, physical structure of the unit, real life situations, etc. may have an effect over the client's behavior in therapeutic environment.

- Maslow in 1968, suggested that the basic needs of an individual have to be fulfilled to move to higher level of functioning.
- Conducive physical facilities have to be provided. For example, privacy physical space that accommodate communal living and facilitates interpersonal interaction and communication.
- Provide democratic environment of self-government. Client participate in decision-making and problem-solving that effect the management of the unit, it will accomplish by attending community meetings organized by residents and staff. All individuals in the group will have equal opportunity in discussions like unit norms, rules, behavioral limits, expectations, etc. in a democratic manner. After discussion by the group, a vote is taken; residents and staff agree to abide by the expressed preference of the majority.
- Unit responsibilities are assigned according to the client's abilities.
- Self-esteem is enhanced by assigning client's responsibilities that promote achievements. Adjustments in assignment are made in a way that preserves self-esteem and progresses the responsibilities and functioning capacity of the client to the previous level.
- A structured program of social and work-related activities is scheduled as a part of treatment program. The therapeutic program include group activities, interpersonal interaction and communication with other individuals are emphasized. Personal problems also will be considered for solution.
- Various group activities may be selected for client with specific needs. For example, exercise group for a person who express anger inappropriately. Assertiveness group for clients with passive aggressive stress management group for anxious clients.
- Change in client's personality and behavior can be affected. New coping strategies and skills will be developed and training will be given in those aspects.
- A structure schedule of activities, which bring change in personality and behavior, can be affected. In the group situation the client is able to practice what he or she has learned to prepare for transition to the general community.

- Community and family are included in the therapeutic program: family members and certain aspects of the community which will affect the client will be included and invited to participate actively in the specific therapeutic groups. For example, sharing, dining, and shopping and or related activities, etc. length of the time will be depend upon client's condition. It facilitates the discharge process and help to prevent the client from becoming too dependent on hospitalization.

FEATURES OF THERAPEUTIC COMMUNITY

- **An informal and communal atmosphere**: The environment is home-like rather than institution.
- **A mutual therapeutic role for residents**: Residents will understand their role and try to understand, how their behavior will be influencing peer group or their surroundings.
- **Sharing decision-making**: Health professional and residents will share their experience and involve actively in decision-making. It may be democratic or hierarchical based on the situation or an event.
- **Residents contribute to the work of maintaining the community activities**: Resident will play a active role, contribute and share with the staff in their activities individualized, unspecified manner voluntarily participates in community activities to meet the need of therapeutic community.
- **Regular community meetings will be held daily**: Where all the member share their information about event and decides the matters which are affecting the community activities and discuss about the problem which will be distributing individual's behavior. Staff members and residents will be encouraged to attend the community meetings following each meeting the staff helps the client to gain insight and the ability to test new behavioral pattern.
- **Staff group therapy sessions**: It can be conducted in each meeting.
- **Staff meeting or review meetings are conducted weekly**: Where the staff will have the opportunity to examine their own responses, expectations and prejudice.
- **Living and learning opportunities or school for living**: It has to be provided to the client within the social living. Where the client can learn to meet the needs and demands of everyday life.
- **Feedback**: It is the fundamental concept in therapeutic community practice.
- **An ideal, dynamic, structured setting will be available in the therapeutic environment**: It includes safe environment, team members and other residents.
- Limits and behavioral expectations are consistently maintained
- Minimizes environmental stressors, develop abilities and strengths, identifies alternate solution of problems.
- To learn about psychodynamics of problems.

- Enhances the resident's responsibilities to work within the social environment by obeying the rules and regulations of society for problem solution with their own efforts.
- Feedback and sharing of responsibilities by the residents is an essential feature of therapeutic community.
- The therapeutic environment is democratic rather than hierarchical rehabilitative rather than custodial permissive instead of limited and controlled.

PRINCIPLES OF THERAPEUTIC COMMUNITY

- *Democratization*: Every member of the community has to share equally in decision-making related to community affairs.
- *Permissiveness*: Every member has to tolerate from one another a wide degree of behavior that may be distressing or deviant from ordinary standards.
- *Communalism*: Free and effective communication and sharing of amenities will be increased thereby hospital authoritativeness and isolation will be reduced.
- *Reality confrontation*: Residents are continuously presented with interpretation of their behavior in order to counteract their tendency to distort, deny or withdraw from their difficulties in getting along with others.
- *Group activity*: Residents and staff members with mutual cooperation, work together to solve the problems of the client. Main aim is solution of problems through group interaction and group activity.
- *Decision-making*: Residents will play active role in deciding their own activities and share equal responsibilities in deciding the activities of community affairs. It will improve the self-confidence of clients.
- *Pattern of attention*: Residents will focus their attention for their needs but also on the needs of other clients.
- The client should have easy approach to interact with the hospital staff members without any inhibition.
- It tries to develop one to one contact.
- Nurse has to be constituent in setting limit and continuous assessment has to be made to evaluate the progress of a client. Needed modified strategies will be implemented in nursing interventions.

PROCEDURE

The morning meeting will be conducted is where all the members of the community analyze the matter of general interest. There is a system of feedback of the event of the previous 24 hours. It is followed by a staff review session, where the main meeting is analyzed and personal contribution and reactions assessed. For example workshop groups, small psychotherapy groups, staff sensitivity groups, assessment sessions.

Immediate business, but the main task is the social analysis of the 'here and now'—What is happening among the members of the groups at that time; always with the eventual aim of increasing the individual awareness and understanding of what he is doing to himself and to other.

TECHNIQUES OF THERAPEUTIC COMMUNITY

Majority of treatments in therapeutic community will takes place in groups as well as in individual; will be used in everyday aspect of community life.

ROLE OF STAFF IN THERAPEUTIC COMMUNITY

- **Participate as a member of the community**: Staff communicates with residents freely and accepts challenges or criticisms with that gap will be removed, a sense of trust and intimacy develops which internalizes the different relationship with authority figures. Staff will act as role model by being open and honest. They will be informally involved and giving training, supervision shows sensitivity toward fulfillment of needs of residents.
- **Maintaining the structure of the community that has to be therapeutic**: Staff will take a lead to re-establish the structure and norms of the community, if need arises and allow the resident to assume their roles and share responsibilities. The structure of the community includes time, place and purpose of different activities defined; the role of different personnel will be prescribed. Clear structures are very important for people with little control over their impulses providing internalizes environment.
- **Provision of living learning experiences**: A wide range of tasks and responsibilities has to be available for the residents, e.g. keeping the community neat and tidy, serving the meals, gardening, etc. whereby the residents will learn to perform different roles and their responsibilities and their self-esteem will be enhanced.
- **Using therapeutic intervention in groups**: Variety of therapeutic intervention like psychoanalysis psychodrama, transactional analysis, cognitive therapy, art therapy, behavioral therapy, etc. is planned for small groups. They provide opportunity for residents to practice these techniques with coresidents, with these techniques, they will be relieved from tensions, worries. Ignore the external criticisms and uses the opportunities in staff meetings, pervasive, therapeutic staff involvement used for the successful treatment of seriously disturbed clients.
- **Maintain external relations**: Staff has to ensure that the unit's role and requirement are well-understood by referrers, colleagues and those who manage parent organization.

ROLES OF INTERDISCIPLINARY TEAM IN THERAPEUTIC COMMUNITY

Psychiatrist

- Serve as a leader of the team
- Diagnosis and treat the cases.

Clinical Psychologist

- Assist in diagnostic process by administering, interpreting and evaluating psychological tests.

Psychiatric Clinical Nurse Specialist

- Conduct psychotherapeutic activities
- Organizes educational programs to the nursing staff
- Provides consultation of services to the nurses, who require assistance in provision of care to the clients.

Mental Health Technician/Psychiatric Aid or Assistant/ Psychiatric Technician

- Assist the clients for fulfillment of their daily living activities.
- Assist the therapeutic team members in implementation of therapeutic activities.

Psychiatric Social Worker

- Concerned with client social needs, e.g. job placement, financial support, location of support, location of community agencies or volunteer.
- Fulfils community and family requirements.
- Assist in conduct of therapeutic activities.
- Follow-up services and continuity of care will be provided.
- Utilizes appropriate community resources.

Occupational Therapist

- Works with the client to develop independent skills.
- Assist the client in performance of daily living activities.
- Gives training for vocational opportunity skills and rehabilitation activities.
- Assist the client to be productive and thereby promotes self-esteem.
- Creative activities and therapeutic skills will be established.

Recreational Therapist

- Assist the clients in redirecting thinking process; rechannelize destructive energy in an appropriate manner.

- Aids the client to spend leisure time in a productive manner by diverting the mind from stress.

Music Therapist

- Encourage the client to express their feelings through music and playing instruments or through dance.

Art Therapist

- Uses the client's creative abilities and encourages expression of emotions and feelings through art works.
- Help the client to analyze their own work in an effort by recognizing and resolving underlying conflicts.

Psychodramatist

- Direct the client to enact by portraying real life situation.
- Some clients are able to act out problem that they are unable to work through in a more traditional manner.

Chaplain

- Identifies and attend spiritual needs of clients and family members by providing spiritual support and comfort.
- Provide counseling services.

ROLE OF NURSE IN THERAPEUTIC COMMUNITY IN A PSYCHIATRY SETTING

Jones has described the nurses responsibilities in three roles.

Authoritarian Role

- Maintaining trusting relationship with the group members.
- The interdisciplinary teamworks within the milieu in a constructive and holistic manner in providing productive and desirable effective treatment.

Social Role

- As a team member, nurse encourages the resident to communicate freely, actively and effectively to participate in discussion.
- Provide moral support to the group members.
- Maintain safe and conflict-free environment for the residents.
- Nurses will encourage their residents to share their responsibilities and participates in group decision making process.
- Assist the client to assume leadership roles by modeling: always give feedback to the client by identifying their abilities and limitations.
- Carrying out supervisory roles.

- Maintain safe environment by not keeping any hazardous material or sharp instruments near the clients.
- Nurses will help the clients to build self-esteem among residents accept the client as a human being, nonjudgmental in nature.

Therapeutic Role

- Establishes therapeutic nurse-client relationship.
- Nurses have to provide the tasks, responsibilities and activities which can be easily accomplished; praise the client for his accomplishment; however it may be very small also.
- Appropriate feedback has to be given whether it may be positive or negative.
- Use confrontation judiciously in a supportive manner.
- Allow the client to identify an alternative approach to the problem solution with the own efforts.
- Client's abilities, strengths are constructively made to influence their own environment, the treatment of others and the organizational structure.
- Psychiatric nurse manipulates the environment to have therapeutic effect. For example, with less stimuli (as calm and quiet) to suit manic residents; provide safe environment in case of high suicidal risk patients; for depressive cases high provoking environmental stimuli will be provided.

RESIDENT ROLES

Active participation and involvement of the resident play a vital role in therapeutic communication treatment. Based on the needs, capabilities and limitations or constraints of an organization, responsibilities will be allotted to the residents.

Therapeutic Roles

Resident's positive feedback always essential to improve other client's behavior. They will give honest feedback to follow residents and support them in times of difficulty by explaining their own experiences in similar situations will have credibility over the therapeutic environment.

Social Role

Living and learning situations provide an opportunities to the residents for introducing the members to the modalities and facilitate interactive communication pattern, overcome isolation feelings.

Decision-making Roles

Residents will encourage taking their decision and helping the coresidents in a number of decisions in their life pattern and organizational activities also will be structured through resident's involvements.

INDIVIDUAL RESPONSIBILITIES

The responsibilities and certain activities will be allotted based on their abilities, interests and organizational requirements. The committee acts as a feedback source for the community, staff and the residents meetings. Leavers group will observe the feeling and problems of residents and guide of residents for further follow-up treatment, the other concern group will help them to understand the aims of the therapeutic community. The staff will be formulating work groups allotting activities like—creative work, pottery, sports and games, gardening, domestic work, cleaning, and maintenance of surroundings.

Nurses are the only healthy personnel, who spend the maximum time with the clients. They assume the responsibility of managing therapeutic milieu through implementing nursing process. Nurses involve in all day to day activities pertaining to client care. Nurses participate in activities to reach the goals of therapy weekly updates and modify treatment plans. Clients will be encouraged to performed treatment plan and daily living activities independently whereby their physiological needs will be met. Nurses make ongoing assessments to plan for provision for assistance or holistic care. Orientation of the client is encouraged; written schedules of activities to be performed by the client will be prepared as a check list, nurses must work with the client to determine methods that result in achievement and provide positive feedback for success. One-to-one relationship has to be established, trust has to be developed. The client will be encouraged to express their emotional feelings and unresolved issues which are creating problems in their personal life.

Nurse is responsible for setting limits on acceptable behavior in understandable terminology, i.e. what behavior are not acceptable and consequences have to be violated these limit must be established, written and carried out the consequences of violation of the established limits is essential, if the learning has to be reinforced. Nurses must be able to assess the learning readiness of the individual client. Nurse must be supportive and encourage the client to become self-reliant, natural social relationships must be fostered, consistent positive outlook is necessary to practice therapeutic environment.

INDICATIONS

- Dependence syndrome
- Depressive disorder
- Neurosis
- Somatoform disorders
- Personality disorders
- Self-harming nature
- Drug abuse
- Violent behavior
- Schizophrenia
- Enduring mental illness.

CONTRAINDICATIONS

- Severe depression
- Acute attack of mania
- Paranoid delusions and paranoid personality.

PARAMETERS OF THERAPEUTIC COMMUNITY

Size of the Unit

The residents in a therapeutic community are 20–30. It allows the group members to experience a number of group situations and memberships and everyone will know each other.

Duration of Treatment

Duration of treatment is 9–18 months, it may be divided into different phases. In acute settings, shorter period and longer period for people with enduring mental illness. For children and adolescents, it may take upto 5 years.

Relations with the Parent's Organizations and Wider Community

It is the vital task for the long-term survival and integrity of a therapeutic community. Managing treatment involves attention, the progress of each resident through the community and the effective functioning of the therapeutic community as a whole.

PHASES OF TREATMENT FOR THE INDIVIDUAL

Therapeutic community works requires a high level of skill and knowledge in a number of areas, together with a well-developed capacity for open honest discussion and reflexion, 20–30 health professional life together for a few days in the residents roles. It provides a valuable opportunity to experience at first-hand the working and impact of this form of treatment.

Starting Treatment

Informal support is given by fellow residents to new resident introduced to the group activities; explain the norm and expectations of the community. New residents in introduction phase will start establishing attachment with coresidents.

Middle Phase

The new residents start to function actively in groups, assisting and helping the coresidents, share their responsibilities. The residents will experience the group situations like dealing with authority fears, feelings like rejections, failure, competition, rivalry, group meetings, staff meetings are conducted where the feelings and experiences and other symptoms of distress. It increases insight and understanding of fellow residents. The resident gradually comes to experience themselves and others differently.

Ending Stage

Residents who complete treatment usually plan their discharge (leaving), fixing the date with the rest of the community. Usually they will develop a strong attachment and dependency on community; hence the Leaver's group will help the residents to overcome the problems of separation and reestablishing life in outside the world. Therapeutic communities also developing aftercare programs, based on their needs, like weekly group sessions or individual support or training, openness, responsibility, rapport, measures for qualitative life, etc. will be inculcated among the residents. The benefits include learning first-hand about the treatment, working as a member of multidisciplinary team, thus gaining experience of institutional dynamics and the way individual react to their wider social networks.

TYPES OF STAFF INVOLVED IN THERAPEUTIC COMMUNITY

Therapeutic community is based on interdisciplinary team treatment (IDT). The interdisciplinary team meets within 48 hours of the admission to determine a comprehensive treatment plan and goal of therapy and to assign intervention responsibilities. All members assign the treatment plan and meet weekly to update the plan as needed.

- Psychiatrist
- Psychiatric clinical nurse
- Clinical psychologist
- Medicosocial worker
- Technical staff
- Support personnel
- Mental health technician
- Occupational therapist
- Recreational therapist
- Art therapist
- Music therapist
- Psychodramatist
- Dietitian
- Chaplain.

THE THERAPEUTIC TOPICS FOR CLIENT EDUCATION

- Way to increase self-esteem
- Stress management techniques
- Anxiety reduction program
- Normal stage of grieving and behavior associated with each stage
- Assertive techniques

- Relaxation techniques
- Effect of substance abuse
- Problem-solving techniques and skills
- Thought stopping and thought switching techniques
- Sex education
- Effective parenting techniques
- Medical diagnosis
- Therapies and follow-up care.

ADVANTAGES OF THERAPEUTIC COMMUNITY

- Initiates good interpersonal relationship among residents and staff members.
- Residents will gain self-confidence.
- Learn to understand themselves and understand others.
- Decide them related to their issues and help others to solve their problems.
- Relearn socialization skills.
- Promote collective thinking and participate in social activities.
- Participate in formulation of rules and regulations of community by actively involving in community meetings.
- Residents learn adoptive acceptable behavior in the therapeutic environment.
- To improve self-esteem.
- Minimize hospital stay and disability.
- To foster therapeutic environment.
- Provide opportunities to participate in community as well as hospital administration.
- Residents will become less dependent and passive.
- Enhances interaction among residents.
- Every individual in the community (staff and residents) will be fully aware of their roles, limitations and responsibilities.
- Residents and staff will be involving in decision making process actively.
- Staff will be able to provide the required information to the residents an job opportunities, half way homes self-help groups.
- In create positive attitude.
- Inculcate productive approach to live happily among residents, as it create homely atmosphere.
- Client becomes less dependent and passive.
- Residents will also making decisions related to ward management and involve in caring other residents.
- Client will be able to learn adaptive, acceptable behavior.
- Resident will be able to control their negative emotions, e.g. hostility and anger.

DISADVANTAGES OF THERAPEUTIC COMMUNITY

- As it is group responsibility, there is a chance nobody will feel a sense of responsibility.
- Individual's needs and concern may not be met.
- Client may find the transition and difficulty to survive within the community.
- Role confusion may be felt for both staff and residents.

ROLE OF THE NURSE IN THERAPEUTIC COMMUNITY

- Providing and maintaining a safe and conflict-free environment through role modeling and group leadership.
- Sharing of responsibilities with parents.
- Encouraging patient to participate in decision-making functions.
- Assisting patients to assume leadership roles.
- Giving feedback.
- Carrying out supervisory functions.

In conclusion, therapeutic community is an approach which is:

- Democratic as opposed to hierarchical.
- Rehabilitative rather than custodial.
- Permissive instead of limited and controlled.

UNIT-III

Somatic (Physical) Therapies

- Electroconvulsive Therapy
- Psychosurgery

Chapter 17 Electroconvulsive Therapy

INTRODUCTION

Electroconvulsive therapy is a type of somatic treatment first introduced by **Bini** and **Cerletti** in April 1938. From 1980 onwards ECT is being considered as a unique psychiatric treatment.

Electroconvulsive therapy is the artificial induction of a grand mal seizures through the application of electrical current to the brain. The stimulus is applied through electrodes that are placed either bilaterally in the frontotemporal region, or unilaterally on the nondominant side. Most client require 6–10 treatment.

HISTORY

The first electroconvulsive therapy was performed in 1938 in Rome by Italian psychiatrists **UGO CERLETTI** and **LUCO BINI**. Electroconvulsive therapy was widely accepted from around 1940–55. This period was followed by a 20 year span during which ECT was considered objectionable. A second peak of acceptance began around 1975 and has been increasing to the present.

DEFINITION

Electroconvulsive therapy is a treatment in which a grand mal seizures through the application of electrical current to the brain while client is under general anesthesia.

TYPES OF ECT

1. *Modified ECT*: Treatment approach whereby pretreatment medications are utilized to initiate treatment.
2. *Unmodified ECT*: Treatment approach without the aid of medication. A concern with this approach in the method is so longer in use.

Parameters of electrical current applied:

Standard dose according to American Psychiatric Association, 1978;
Voltage— 70–120 Volt
Duration— 0.7–1.5 second

TYPES OF SEIZURES PRODUCED

1. Grand mal seizures— Tonic phase lasting for 10–15 sec.
2. Clonic Phase— Lasting for 30–60 seconds.

PROCEDURE

Electroconvulsive therapy involve the passage of an electrical stimulus of 70–150 Volts to the brain for 0.7–1.5 sec to procedure a grand mal seizures. Seizure induction is necessary to achieve the therapeutic effect, which is thought to be the result of an alteration in the postsynaptic response to the neurotransmitters in the central nervous system.

The client receives atropine sulfate subcutaneously before the procedure and at the beginning of the treatment as intravenous dose of sodium pentothal. Electrode jelly is applied bilaterally to the temples or unilaterally to the padded electrodes. An airway or soft mouth gag is put in the client's mouth to present tongue bite. Succinylcholine is also administered. The resulting grand mal seizure closely resembles a tonic phase (tightening of muscles) for approximately 10 seconds and a clonic phase (rhythmic movements of the muscles) for 30 seconds. The movements are slight and often limited to plantar flexion of the feet, followed by rhythmic twitching to the toes. The seizure is accompanied by a short period of apnea and then stertorous (snoring like) respiration by mechanical means if necessary. Usually the client sleep for 5–10 minutes after seizures, slowly awakens and does not remember the treatment.

MECHANISM OF ACTION

The exact mechanism of action is not known. One hypothesis states that is possible affects the catecholamine pathway between encephalon and limbic system, also involves the hypothalamus.

FREQUENCY AND TOTAL NUMBER OF ECT

Frequency— 3 times per week or as indicated.
Total no.— 6 –10 upto 25 may be preferred as indicated.

INDICATIONS

A. *Major depression*: With suicidal risk, with stupor, poor intake of food and fluid, melancholia, psychotic features, unsatisfactory responses to drug or where drugs are indicated or have serious side effects.
B. *Severe catatonia*: With suicidal risk, with stupor, poor intake of food and fluid unsatisfactory responses to drugs or where drugs are indicated or have serious side effects.
C. *Severe psychosis*: With risk of suicide, homicide or danger of physical assult, depressive features with unsatisfactory response to drug therapy, or when drugs are contraindicated or have serious side effects.

D. *Organic mental disorders*: Organic mood disorder, organic psychosis.

Other Indications

ECT is preferred to antidepressants therapy in some cases, such as, for client with cardiac disease, when tricycles are contraindicated because heart failure, and for pregnant women in which antidepressants place the feature at risk for congenital defects.

CONTRAINDICATIONS

There are no absolute indications to ECT, however, relative contraindications are—

- Increased intracranial pressure
- Cerebrovascular accident
- Spaceoccupying intracranial lesions
- Cervical injury or problem
- Head injury
- Recent myocardial infarctions.

RISK ASSOCIATED WITH ECT

1. Mortality—Death is rare and usually related to cardiovascular complications
2. Cognitive impairment, memory loss has both retrograde components
3. Brain damage.

COMPLICATION OF ECT

With threatening complication of ECT does not cause any brain damage fracture can sometimes occur in elderly patient with osteoporosis. In patient with a history of heart disease. Dysthymias and respiratory arrest may occur.

SIDE EFFECTS OF ECT

- Memory impairment
- Drowsiness, confusion and restlessness
- Poor concentration and anxiety
- Headache, weakness, fatigue, backache, and muscle ache
- Dryness of mouth, palpitation, nausea, and vomiting
- Unsteady gait
- Tongue bite and incontinence.

ECT TEAM

- Psychiatrist
- Anesthesiologist
- Trained nurses
- Assistants.

Treatment facilities— There should be suite from 3 rooms.

1. A pleasant comfortable waiting room or pre-ECT room.
2. ECT room— In which should be equipped with ECT machine and accessories, an anesthetic appliance, suction apparatus, facemasks, oxygen cylinder with adjustable flow valves, curved tongue and emergency drug, there should be immediate access to a defibrilization.
3. A well-equipped recovery room.

ROLE OF NURSES

Preprocedure

- Detailed medical and psychiatric history, including the history of allergies.
- Assessment of patient and family knowledge of indication, side effects, therapeutic effect and risk associated with ECT.
- An informed consent should be taken, allay any found fear and anxieties regarding the procedure.
- Assess baseline vital signs.
- Patient should be on empty stomach for 46 hours prior to ECT.
- Withhold night doses of drug which increase seizures threshold like lorazepam, barbiturates and anticonvulsants.
- Withhold any medication in the morning.
- Head shampooing in the morning since oil causes impedance of passages of electricity to brain.
- Any jewelry, prosthesis, dentures, contact lenses, metallic objects and tight clothing should be removed from the patient body.
- Empty bowel and bladder just before ECT.
- Administration of 0.6 mg atropine IM or SC 30 miniutes before ECT or IV just before ECT.

Intraprocedure Care

- Place the patient comfortably on the ECT table in the supine position.
- Stay with the patient to allay anxiety and fear.
- Assist in administrating the anesthetic agent thiopentothal sodium 3–5 mg/kg body weight and muscle relaxant succinylcholine 1mg/kg body weight.
- Since the muscle relaxant paralyzes all muscle including respiratory muscles patient airway should be ensure and ventilatory support should be started.
- Mouth gag should be inserted to prevent possible tongue bite.
- The place of electrode placement should be cleaned with normal saline or 25% bicarbonate solution or a conducting gel applied.
- Monitor voltage intensity and duration of electrical stimulus given.

- Monitor seizure activity using cuff method.
- 100% oxygen should be provided.
- During seizure monitor vital signs ECG, oxygen saturation, EEG, etc.
- Record the findings and medicine given in the patient's charts.

Postprocedure Care

- Monitor vital signs.
- Continue oxygen till spontaneous respiration starts.
- Assess for postictal confusion and restlessness.
- Take safety precaution to prevent injury (side-lying position and suctioning to prevent aspiration of secretion, use of side rails to prevent falls.
- If severe postictal confusion and restlessness, IV diazepam may be administered.
- Reorient the patient after recovery and stay with him until fully oriented.
- Document any findings or relevant in the patient record.

GUIDELINES FOR TREATMENT

Experts disagree on whether ECT is an appropriate first-line treatment or if it should be reserved for patients who have not responded to other interventions such as medication and psychotherapy.

The *American Psychiatric Association* (APA) 2001 guidelines give the primary indications for ECT among patients with depression as a lack of response to, or intolerance of, *antidepressant* medications; a good response to previous ECT; and the need for a rapid and definitive response (e.g. because of *psychosis* or a risk of *suicide*). The decision to use ECT depends on several factors, including the severity and chronicity of the depression, the likelihood that alternative treatments would be effective, the patient's preference and capacity to consent, and a weighing of the risks and benefits.

Some guidelines recommend *cognitive behavioral therapy* or other *psychotherapy* before ECT is used. However, treatment resistance is widely defined as lack of therapeutic response to two antidepressants at adequate doses for an adequate duration and with good compliance. The APA states that at times patients will prefer to receive ECT over alternative treatments, but commonly the opposite will be the case.

The APA ECT guidelines state that severe *major depression* with psychotic features, manic delirium, or *catatonia* are conditions where there is a clear consensus favoring early ECT. The *UK's National Institute for Health and Clinical Excellence* (NICE) guidelines recommend ECT for patients with severe depression, *catatonia*, or prolonged or severe *mania*. Indeed, the updated (2009). NICE guidelines for depression also provide for the use of maintenance ECT (where ECT is given at longer intervals to prevent relapse), although the guidance stresses the need for further study. The 2001 APA guidelines also support the use of ECT for relapse prevention.

The 2001 APA ECT guidelines say that ECT is rarely used as a first-line treatment for *schizophrenia* but is considered after unsuccessful treatment with antipsychotic medication, and may also be considered in the treatment of patients with *schizoaffective* or *schizophreniform* disorder. The 2003 NICE ECT guidelines do not recommend ECT for schizophrenia, and this has been supported by *meta-analytic* evidence showing no or little benefit versus *placebo*, or in combination with *antipsychotic* drugs, including clozapine.

The NICE 2003 guidelines state that doctors should be particularly cautious when considering ECT treatment for women who are *pregnant* and for older or younger people, because they may be at higher risk of complications with ECT. The 2001 APA ECT guidelines say that ECT may be safer than alternative treatments in the infirm elderly and during pregnancy, and the 2000 APA depression guidelines stated that the literature supports the safety for mother and *fetus*, as well as the efficacy during pregnancy.

Adverse Effects

Aside from effects in the brain, the general physical risks of ECT are similar to those of brief *general anesthesia*; the United States' Surgeon General's report says that there are 'no absolute health *contraindications*' to its use. Immediately following treatment the most common adverse effects are confusion and memory loss. The state of confusion usually disappears after a few hours. It can be tolerated by pregnant women who are not suffering major complications. It can be used with diabetic or obese patients, and with caution in those whose cancers are in remission or under control. It can be used in some immunocompromised patients. It must be used very cautiously in people with epilepsy or other neurological disorders because by its nature it provokes small tonic-clonic seizures, and so would likely not be given to a person whose epilepsy is not well-controlled. Some patients experience muscle soreness after ECT. This is due to the muscle relaxants given during the procedure and rarely due to muscle activity. The death rate due to ECT is around 4 per 100,000 procedures.

Effects on memory

It is the purported effects of ECT on long-term memory that give rise to much of the concern surrounding its use. The acute effects of ECT can include *amnesia*, both retrograde (for events occurring before the treatment) and anterograde (for events occurring after the treatment). However, the vast majority of these effects are short-lived. Memory loss and confusion are more pronounced with bilateral electrode placement rather than unilateral, and with outdated sine-wave rather than briefpulse currents. The vast majority of modern treatment uses brief pulse currents. Research by *Harold Sackeim* has shown that excessive current causes more risk for memory loss, and using right-sided electrode placement may reduce verbal memory disturbance.

Retrograde amnesia is most marked for events occurring in the weeks or months before treatment, with one study showing that although some people lose memories from years prior to treatment, recovery of such memories was 'virtually complete' by seven months posttreatment, with the only enduring loss being memories in the weeks and months prior to the treatment. *Anterograde memory loss* is usually limited to the time of treatment itself or shortly afterwards. In the weeks and months following ECT these memory problems gradually improve, but some people have persistent losses, especially with bilateral ECT.

Some studies have found that patients are often unaware of cognitive deficits induced by ECT. For example, in June 2008, a Duke University study was published assessing the neuropsychological effects and attitudes in patients after ECT. Forty-six patients participated in the study, which involved neuropsychological and psychological testing before and after ECT. The study documented substantial cognitive impairment after ECT on a variety of memory tests, including 'verbal memory for word lists and prose passages and visual memory of geometric designs'. The study further found that a significant number of patients believed that their memory had improved after ECT despite the fact that neuropsychological testing clearly showed the opposite. As stated by the researchers, 'Indeed, there was a slight trend towards improved memory functioning, despite the objective neuropsychological data indicating significantly lower recognition and delayed recall'. Based on their findings, the authors issued the following recommendation:

When ECT is provided to adolescents, the potential impact of such cognitive changes should be discussed with the patients and their parents or guardians in terms of implications for not only the patient's emotional functioning but cognitive functioning as well, particularly upon his or her academic performance. In summary, we argue that an individual cost-benefit analysis should be made in light of the implications of the potential benefits versus costs of ECT upon improving emotional functioning and the impact that potential memory changes may have on real-world functioning and quality of life.

Effects in pregnancy

If steps are taken to decrease potential risks, ECT is generally accepted to be relatively safe during all trimesters of pregnancy, particularly when compared to pharmacological treatments. Suggested preparation for ECT during pregnancy includes a *pelvic examination*, discontinuation of nonessential *anticholinergic* medication, uterine *to codynamometry*, intravenous hydration, and administration of a nonparticulate antacid. During ECT, elevation of the pregnant woman's right hip, external fetal cardiac monitoring, *intubation*, and avoidance of excessive *hyperventilation* are recommended. Much of the medical literature in this area is composed of case studies of single or twin pregnancies, and although some have reported serious complications, the majority have found ECT to be safe. ECT is not performed on the fetus.

ADMINISTRATION

Informed consent is sought before treatment. Patients are informed about the risks and benefits of the procedure. Patients are also made aware of risks and benefits of other treatments and of not having the procedure done at all. Depending on the jurisdiction the need for further inputs from other medical professionals or legal professionals may be required. ECT is usually given on an inpatient basis. Prior to treatment a patient is given a short-acting anesthetic such as *methohexital, etomidate,* or *thiopental,* a muscle relaxant such as *suxamethonium* (succinylcholine), and occasionally *atropine* to inhibit salivation (Fig. 17.1).

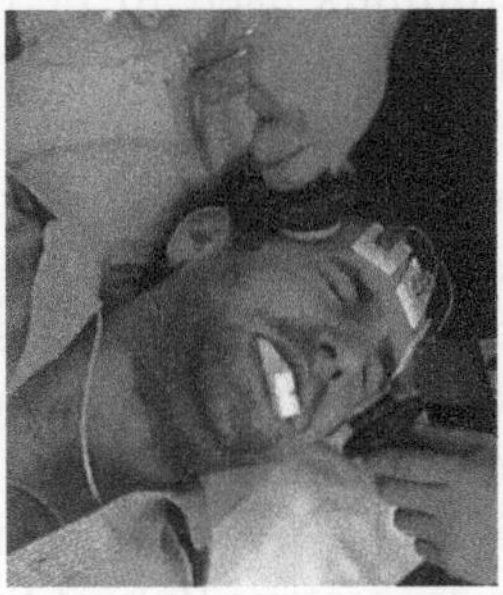

Figure 17.1: Placement of electrodes

MECHANISM OF ACTION

The aim of ECT is to induce a therapeutic clonic *seizure* (a seizure where the person loses consciousness and has convulsions) lasting for at least 15 seconds. Although a large amount of research has been carried out, the exact mechanism of action of ECT remains elusive. The main reasons for this are that the human brain cannot be studied directly before and after ECT and therefore scientists rely on animal models of depression and ECT, with major limitations. While animal models are acknowledged to model merely aspects of depressive illness, human and animal brains are very similar at a molecular level, enabling detailed study of the molecular mechanisms involved in ECT.

Involuntary ECT

Procedures for involuntary ECT vary from country to country depending on local *mental health laws.* Legal proceedings are required in some countries, while in others ECT is seen as another form of treatment that may be given involuntarily as long as legal conditions are observed.

Involuntary electroshock contravenes the principle of autonomy in *medical ethics*. The maxim of autonomy is 'Voluntas aegroti suprema lex'. This rule states that the will of the patient is supreme. It implies that a patient has the right to consent to, or to refuse a medical treatment, such as ECT. Persons considered not to be of sound mind are in many jurisdictions considered incapable of giving true consent. In such a case, the patient's 'assent' may be sought; opinions are divided as to whether this should be routinely done, or whether a patient who is not competent to consent to therapy should retain the right to refuse it.

ECT Machines

Most modern ECT machines deliver a brief-pulse current, which is thought to cause fewer cognitive effects than the sine-wave currents which were originally used in ECT. A small minority of psychiatrists in the USA still use sine-wave stimuli. Sine-wave is no longer used in the UK or Ireland. Typically, the electrical stimulus used in ECT is about 800 *milliamps* and has upto several hundred *watts*, and the current flows for between one and 6 seconds. In the USA, ECT machines are manufactured by two companies, Somatics, which is owned by psychiatrists Richard Abrams and Conrad Swartz, and *Mecta*. The *Food and Drug Administration* has classified the devices used to administer ECT as *Class III medical devices*. Class III is the highest-risk class of medical devices. In the UK, the market for ECT machines was long monopolized by Ectron Ltd, although in recent years some hospitals have started using American machines. Ectron Ltd was set up by psychiatrist Robert Russell, who together with a colleague from the Three Counties Asylum, Bedfordshire, invented the Page-Russell technique of intensive ECT.

Both electrodes can be placed one on the same side of the patient's head. This is known as unilateral ECT (Fig. 17.2). Unilateral ECT is used first to minimize side effects (memory loss). When electrodes are placed on both sides of the head, this is known as bilateral ECT. In bifrontal ECT, an uncommon variation, the electrode position is somewhere between

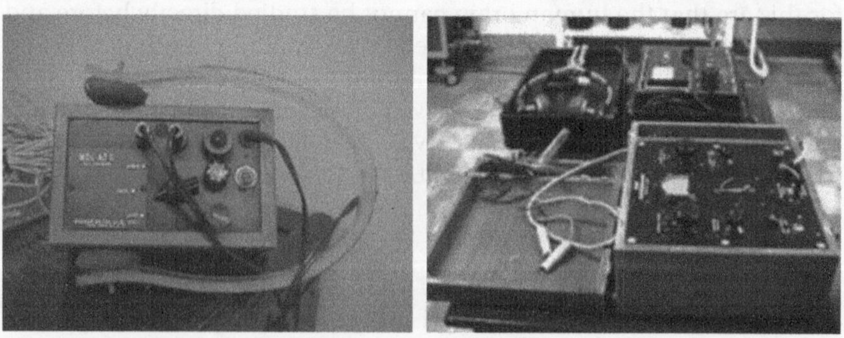

Figure. 17.2: ECT machines

bilateral and unilateral. Unilateral is thought to cause fewer cognitive effects than bilateral but is considered less effective. In the USA most patients receive bilateral ECT. In the UK almost all patients receive bilateral ECT.

The electrodes deliver an electrical stimulus. The stimulus levels recommended for ECT are in excess of an individual's *seizure threshold*: about one and a half times *seizure threshold* for bilateral ECT and upto 12 times for unilateral ECT. Below these levels treatment may not be effective in spite of a seizure, while doses massively above threshold level, especially with bilateral ECT, expose patients to the risk of more severe *cognitive impairment* without additional therapeutic gains. Seizure threshold is determined by trial and error (dose titration). Some psychiatrists use dose titration, some still use 'fixed dose' (that is, all patients are given the same dose) and others compromise by roughly estimating a patient's threshold according to age and sex. Older men tend to have higher thresholds than younger women, but it is not a hard and fast rule, and other factors, for example drugs, affect seizure threshold.

Chapter 18 Psychosurgery

INTRODUCTION

It was developed by Ega Moniz in 1936. It is used to affect the patient's psychological state, modification of the disturbed behavior, thought content or mood.

DEFINITION

Psychosurgery is defined by APA'S taskforce as, a surgical treatment or intervention, to severe fiber connecting one part of brain with another or to remove, destroy or stimulate brain tissue with intent of modifying behavior, thought or mood disturbances, for which there is no underlying organic pathology (i.e. the disturbance is functional).

INDICATIONS

1. Chronic severe psychiatric illness, e.g. depression, OCD, anxiety, schizophrenia with severe depression, uncontrolled aggressive behavior
2. Chronic duration of illness of about 10 years
3. Persistent emotional distress
4. Failure to respond all other therapies
5. High risk of suicide.

MECHANISM OF ACTION

Limbic system is closely linked with normal and abnormal emotional reaction. Limbic system is closely connected with frontal and temporal lobes, midbrain and other part of the brain by many connecting fibers.

The aim of psychosurgery is to produce surgical lesion in carefully selected part of limbic system and/or its connecting fibers.

PAPEZ CIRCUIT

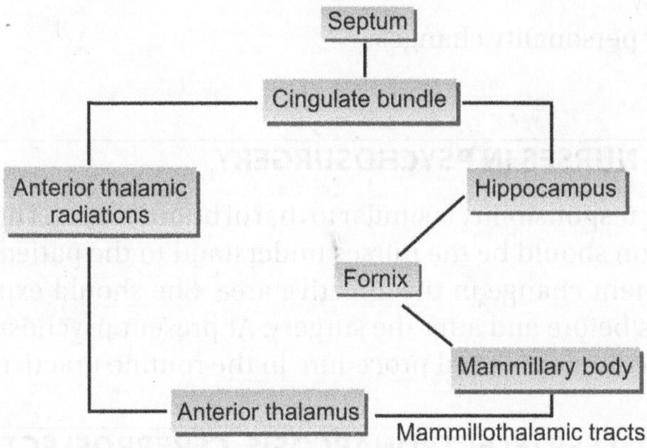

TECHNIQUES AND TYPES OF OPERATION

Before any procedure, an informed consent must be obtained by the neurosurgeon and the treatment team.

Current all techniques use stereotactic methods.

The available prokedures are:

- Bimedial leukotomy
- Prefrontal leukotomy
- Orbital undercutting
- Rostal leukotomy
- Anterior or posterior cingulotomy.

The lesion is produced by electrocoagulation, ultrasonic method, Yttrium 90 seeds or laser.

THE CURRENTLY EMPLOYED PROCEDURES

1. *Stereotactic subacute tractotomy*: A large subcaudate lesion is produced. It is recommended for severe anxiety and schizoaffective disorder.
2. *Stereotactic limbic leukotomy*: A small subcaudate lesion is made in addition to a lesion cingulated bundle. It is used for treatment of OCD and schizophrenia.
3. *Amygdalotomy*: This is used for severe, pathological uncontrolled and Interactable aggression associated with neuropsychiatric disorders.

SIDE EFFECTS

- Poor impulse control
- Psychopathic disorder
- Drug addiction, alcoholism
- Diffuse brain damage and cerebrovascular disease.

COMPLICATIONS

1. Epilepsy
2. Lasting personality changes
3. Apathy.

ROLE OF NURSES IN PSYCHOSURGERY

The nursing responsibility is similar to that of brain surgery. The important consideration should be the nurses understand to the patient who have this permanent change in the affective area. She should explain this to the relatives before and after the surgery. At present psychosurgery is an extreme uncommonly used procedure in the routine practice in India.

ELECTROSLEEP (ELECTRONARCOSIS, CEREBROELECTROTHERAPY—CET)

This techniques involves the use of a low amplitude pulsating direct current which is applied to the forehead and/or mastoid area. No drug or anesthetics are used. The current procedures a tingling sensation in the skin and appear to induce a state of relaxation for 30 minutes or 1 hour.

Indication

- Anxiety (Particularly chronic unremitting anxiety).

MEGA VITAMIN THERAPY

High dose of Vit B_{12} or nicotinic acid is administered. Other combination such as, Vit C or/ and Vit E are also used.

A lot of improvement in the method of treatment used for mentally ill. Planned research have to be continued in the area to find out method of treatment to cure mental illness.

UNIT-IV
Activity Therapy

- Occupational Therapy
- Recreational Therapy
- Relaxation Therapy
- Educational Therapy
- Bibliotherapy
- Play Therapy
- Music Therapy
- Dance Therapy
- Art Therapy
- Light Therapy
- Color Therapy
- Aromatherapy
- Spiritual Therapy

Chapter 19 Occupational Therapy

INTRODUCTION

Occupational therapy has been described as an active method of treatment with a profound psychological justification (Clark 1963). The essence of occupational therapy lies in the use of activities of every description as treatment medium, with a minimum aim of complete rehabilitation. It is the application of goal-oriented purposeful activity in the assessment and the treatment of individuals with psychological, physical or developmental disabilities. Therapist will utilize proper use of time in some useful and meaningful goal-oriented activities, whereby the client can practice his social communication and interpersonal skills to lead productive life after discharge.

Historical background—In 1752 the Pennsylvania Hospital, Philadelphia, was established in USA, where the use of occupation as treatment for mentally ill continued to develop until the Civil war in 1860.

- In December 1914 architect George Edward Boston attended a meeting of hospital workers and the Massachusetts state board of Insanity (Hopkins 1983). During his own recent illness he had received.
- At a meeting in March 1917 held at consolidation house, Clifton Springs, New York, the National Society for the promotion of occupational therapy was formed, incooperated and charted under the laws of district of Columbia. This body helps its first AGM in September 1917 in New York city.
- William Dunton established the first in Maryland and a Pattern of National Body were formed. This remains the basic pattern for 'The American Occupational Therapy Association (AOTA)', as it has been known since 1923.
- Occupational therapy for a modern psychiatric hospital was introduced into Scotland at Gartnavel Royal Mental Hospital in 1919 by Dr DK Henderson, later known as professor Sir David Henderson.
- The first school of occupational therapy was at Darset House in UK was found in 1930 under Dr Carson's inspiration and with tebbit as its first principal.

DEFINITIONS

1. *According to Read and Sanderson, 1980*: Any activity which engages a person's resources of time and energy and is composed of skills and values.

2. *According to Jhonson, 1973*: Any goal directed meaningful activity to the individual and providing feedback to his worth and value as an individual about his interrelatedness to others.

AIMS

1. Social aims—
- To give residents break from institutional life.
- To teach clients to find their way around the locality and use a community facility.
- To promote communication (including the use of sign language).
- To develop a sense of belong by increasing group cohesion.

2. Physical aims—
- To improve coordination and spatial awareness.
- To improve general physical condition and increase cardiovascular fitness.
- To develop strength and suppleness and to improve posture and gait.

3. Personal aims—
- To improve mood and reduce anxiety.
- To provide an outlet for aggressive impulses.
- To improve confidence and enhance self-image.
- To encourage independent personal care (especially dressing and grooming).
- To provide opportunities for clients to face challenges and achieves success.

OBJECTIVES

1. To develop, relearn, improve and maintain the social, communicational and occupational skills to achieve high level of competency for satisfactory performance of their roles.
2. Meet the client needs in a socially acceptable approved manner.
3. Improve the role performance of the clients.
4. Improve the quality of life.
5. To take control over their lives and overcome their own disabilities.
6. Engage the client in useful constructive activities.
7. Attain the highest functional ability.
8. Teach the client self-care activities.
9. Maintain life activities after discharge.
10. Attain and satisfy needs of the client by giving them love and affection and making them feel accepted by all those around them.
11. Improve the self-esteem and self-confidence.
12. Overcome disabilities.
13. Modify the maladaptive behavior.
14. Improves the socialization and cooperation along with others.
15. Re-establish social relationships between the client and other societal members and allowing them to work along with other group members.

16. Prevent hospitalization for chronic cases.
17. Improve the attention and concentration, time and quality work of the client.
18. Remove or minimize behaviors that interfere with occupational performance.
19. Improve physical coordination and spastial awareness.
20. Improve general physical condition, e.g. cardiovascular fitness, posture, gait, and moods.
21. Reduce anxiety.
22. Provide on outlet for emotional impulses, e.g. aggressive.
23. Develop more healthy and integrated ego.
24. To assist the client in making a transition from sick role to becoming a contributing member of the society.
25. To assist in diagnostic and personality evaluation.
26. To enhance psychotherapy and other psychotherapeutic measures (the activity prescribed for the client often provides a nonverbal means for the client to express and resolve his feelings).
27. Create variety of interests and facilities constructive work, makes the client to understand their role in the work.
28. Develop a spirit of hope, faith and a sense of accomplishment so that client can work for their future after discharge.
29. Correct psychopathology.
30. Facilitates personality integration.
31. Develops more realistic view of the self in relation to others.
32. To improve client perception, cognition, coordination, conceptual and formal discrimination.
33. Provide a supported stepping stone to go back to mainstream work.
34. Motivate the client in structured program of activity, may distract them from their symptoms.
35. Engage their leisure time in useful activities.
36. Improve confidence and self-image.
37. Restore the lost skills, e.g. after recovery from head injury, practicing the precision, skillful movements.
38. Provide opportunities for client to face challenges and achieves success.
39. Enhance sensory integration, normalize motor and perceptual responses.
40. Strengthen ego defenses.
41. Teach the client the skills needed to cope outside hospital and then gradually reintroduce them to life in the community.

GOALS

The main goal is to enable the attend to achieve a healthy balance of occupations through the development of skills that will allow him to function at the level satisfactory to himself and others.

The goal of occupational therapy activities is to alleviate physical and cognitive disabilities by emphasizing performance, so that children and adults can lead fulfilling lives. The disabilities addressed may be congenital or may have resulted from accident-related injuries. Occupational activities are frequently implemented with the elderly when there is general physical and mental decline due to the aging process. Working with crafts, training in daily skills, and vocational training are all activities that may be performed in occupational therapy.

While the kind and scope of occupational therapy activities has expanded over the years, arts and crafts was the medium through which therapists originally sought to facilitate adaptation and even cure for physical and psychological disabilities. This curative effect is thought to generalize to society. In any case, for many patients, arts and crafts remain an integral part of occupational therapy.

SETTINGS

Occupational therapy is provided to children, adolescents, adults and elderly patients these programs are offered in—

- Psychiatric hospitals
- Schools
- Nursing homes
- Rehabilitation center
- Special schools
- Community group homes
- Day care centers
- Half way homes
- Deaddiction centers
- Psychiatric institutions
- Outreach centers
- Group centers
- Sheltered workshops and clinics
- Handicapped homes
- Industrial health units.

ORGANIZATIONS OF OCCUPATIONAL THERAPY

- Assessment of needs
- Fixing up of specific objectives
- Choosing right type of work and play
- Incentives
- Motivation and training
- Evaluation of improvement
- Rehabilitation.

ORGANIZATIONS OF OCCUPATIONAL THERAPEUTIC TEAM

- Psychiatrist
- Psychologist

- Psychosocial worker
- Psychiatric nurse
- Occupational therapist
- Recreational therapist
- Physiotherapist
- Speech therapist
- Art therapist
- Social worker
- Family and friends.

ADVANTAGES

1. Help to develop social skills and provide an outlet for self-expression
2. Strengthens ego defenses
3. Develop a more realistic view of the self in relation to others.

POINTS TO BE KEPT IN MIND

- The client should be involved as much as possible in selecting the activity.
- Select an activity that interests or has potential to interest him.
- The activity should utilize the client strengths and abilities.
- The activity should be short duration to foster a feeling of accomplishment.
- If possible, the select activity should provide some new experience for the client.

TYPES OF ACTIVITIES

A. Divertional activities: These activities are used to divert one's thoughts from life stresses or to fill time, e.g. organized games.
B. Therapeutic activities: These activities are used to attain a specific care plan or goal, e.g. basket making, carpentry.
C. Remedial activities: Emphasized on rehabilitation aspect, e.g. skill/ motor training-embroidery, gardening.
D. Individual training.
E. Group training.

PURPOSES

- Stimulates spontaneity
- Stimulates freedom of movements
- Stimulate competitiveness
- Stimulate excitement
- Overcome anxiety, frustration and fear.

PRINCIPLE

- Involve the client in selection of the activity—
  1. Selection the activities based on interests, IQ levels, strength and abilities of the clients.
  2. Utilizes the client resources.
  3. Start the point the client is at and progress slowly, let him make the pace.
  4. Short duration activities are selected to foster a sense of accomplishment feelings.
  5. Provide ample reinforcement for even small achievement.
  6. The selected activity has to give a new experience for the client.

PROCESS OF INTERVENTION (FIG. 19.1)

It consists of six stages—

1. Initial evaluation of what patient can do and cannot do in a variety of situations over a period of time.
2. Development of immediate and long-term goals by the patient and therapist together. Goals should be concrete and measurable so that it is easy to see when they have been attained.
3. Development of therapy plan with planned intervention.
4. Implementation of the plan and monitoring the progress. The plan is followed until the first evaluation of satisfactory it is continued or altered if not.
5. Review meetings with patient and all the staff involved in treatment.
6. Setting further goals when immediate goals have been achieved, modifying the treatment program as relevant.
7. Functional regularity are established in the client's mind and they feel there is worthwhile and lead a pleasant life.

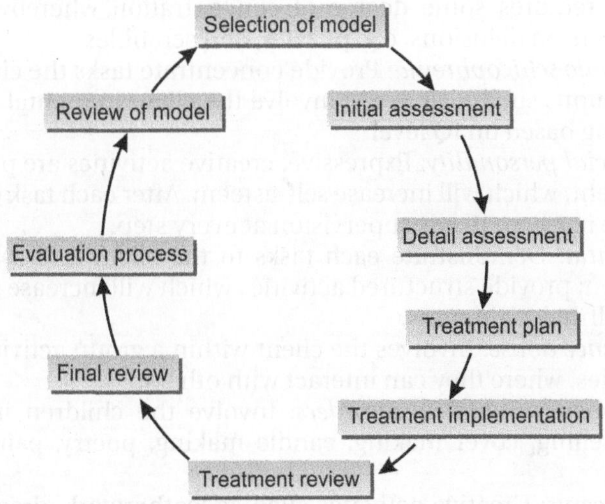

Figure 19.1: The occupational therapy process (Model)

The Quality Assurance Circle of Activity

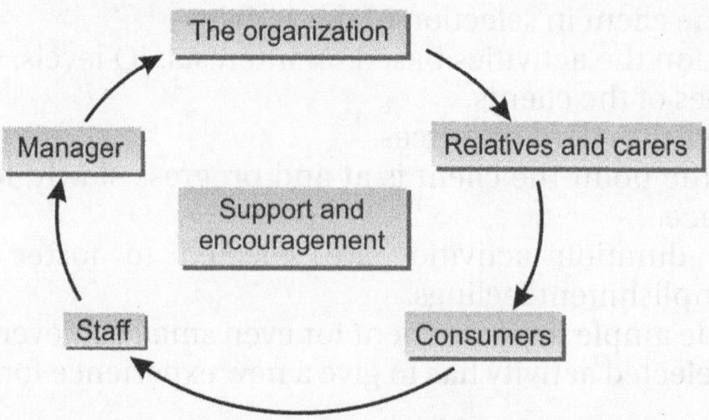

INDICATIONS

A. *Depression*: It makes the clients to sit and watch initially in order to socialize them to feel to perform certain activities. Provide positive reinforcement after each achievement, e.g. crafts, gardening, mowing lawn, and weeding.

B. *Chronic schizophrenia*: Sensory integration approach, e.g. throwing the ball overhead, ducking under nets, marching, and skipping. Protective methods, e.g. writing story, drawing, and asking them to write whatever comes to the mind.

C. *Anxiety disorder*: Simple concrete task with not more than 3 or 4 steps that can be learnt quickly, e.g. washing, mopping, sweeping, and weeding.

D. *Manic disorders*: Noncompetitive activities that allow the energy use and expression of feelings, limited activities, client has to work away from distractions, e.g. mental work, clay molding, and raking grass.

E. *Paranoid schizophrenia*: Noncompetitive, solitary meaningful tasks which requires some degree of concentration whereby they can deviate from delusions, e.g. puzzles, and scrabbles.

F. *Catatonic schizophrenia*: Provide concentrate tasks the client needs continuous supervision, e.g. involve the client in mental work, clay molding based on IQ level.

G. *Antisocial personality*: Expressive, creative activities are provided to the client, which will increase self-esteem. After each task completes ensure it. Client needs supervision at every step.

H. *Dementia*: Demonstrate each tasks to the client and ask them to repeat it; provide structured activities which will increase self-worth and self-belongingness.

I. *Substance abuse*: Involves the client within a group activities/social activities, where they can interact with others.

J. *Childhood psychiatric disorders*: Involve the children in playing, story telling, cover making, candle making, poetry, painting, and music.

K. *Adolescents*: Creative activities such as leatherwork, drawing, and painting.

L. *Mental retardation*: Repetitive work assignments, are ideals, provide reinforcement after each achievement, e.g. cover making, candle making, packaging goods, etc.

WHEN TO REFER A PATIENT TO PSYCHIATRIC OT

Patients should be referred whose daily living skills are impaired, due to:
- Treatment noncompliance or resistance
- Severe lack of motivation or investment
- Depressive symptoms: Anhedonia, apathy, isolation, social avoidance, indifference, vegetative state, and crying
- Adjustment reaction: Depression, ruminating, reaction out of character for patient or out of proportion to physical insult, anger, hostility, blaming, and treatment refusal
- Anxiety prohibiting function
- Cognitive impairment due to psychosis
- Chronic pain/behavioral maladaptation.

MEDICAL DIAGNOSES WITH POTENTIAL FOR PSYCHOLOGICAL SEQUELAE INCLUDE

- Leukemia
- Carcinoma
- COPD
- Transplant
- Colorectal dysfunction
- Amputation
- Cardiac disorders
- AIDS
- Inflammatory disorders
- Postconcussional syndrome
- ESRD.

Type of Services Planned

1. Relaxation techniques, e.g. physiological methods, medication techniques, hypnotic suggestions, swimming, dance technique, and exercises— walking, running, and jogging.
2. Task-oriented activities, e.g. mother crafts, kitchen work, cover making, play activity, bakery, and pantry.
3. Work adjustment programs/productive work, e.g. child rearing practices, handloom section, soap making, basket making, carpentry work, plastic moulding, printing, and stationary.
4. Prevocational activities, e.g. jumping, skipping, hopping, crawling, rolling, and throw ball.
5. Design fabrication, e.g. weaving, mat making, doll preparation, sewing, leather work, and wood work.

6. Therapeutic exercises.
7. Adaptation to physical environment.
8. Patient or family education, counseling for community reentry by discharge planning and advices.
9. Group participation activities.

ROLE OF NURSE IN OCCUPATIONAL THERAPY

1. Coordinate with other team members in diagnosing the abilities, strengthen, talents, interests IQ levels of the client and in selecting the activity for a specific client.
2. Provide a series of graded experiences to the client, e.g. observing the demonstration of any activity to more direct and active experiences.
3. Educate the client to develop specific new skills.
4. Encourages socialization of the client and exhibits, positive interest.
5. Guides the client in information of new hobbies by strengthening the abilities of the client.
6. Support, supervises and cooperates the patient in implementation of work-related activities.
7. Appreciates, if the client performs any approved activity.
8. After token of econony, each accomplishment of the work.
9. Help the client to develop independent living skills.
10. Approaches community agencies for job placement of the clients, after discharge.
11. Needed guidance will be provided to family members.
12. Friendly in nature, counsel the client in approved social activities.
13. Assist in developing good social interaction and relationship.
14. Never criticizes the client, when he is performing any activity.
15. Provides continuous, constant encouragement and support.
16. Assist in psychosocial productiveness of the client.

List of Activities Guided by the Nurse in the Hospital Situation

1. Activities in the ward— Assist in bed making, dusting, cleaning furniture, and washing floors and clothes.
2. Activities in library— Book binding, book keeping, issues books, maintaining records, etc.
3. Activities in workshops/crafts, e.g. cane works, basket making, knitting, washing, preparation of decorating pieces, toys and dolls, candles, greeting cards, envelopes, paper bags, etc.
4. Gardening and assisting in poultry farms or animals husbandry.
5. Maintaining hygiene of kitchen, assist in diet, distribution to the client in ward, preparing tea, coffee, toasts, meals, etc.

Chapter 20 Recreational Therapy

INTRODUCTION

Recreation is a form of activity therapy used in most psychiatric settings. It is a planned therapeutic activity that enables people with limitations to engage in recreational experiences. It assist the client in making a transition from sick role to becoming a contributing a member of the society.

Recreation therapy is the provision of treatment, leisure education and recreational services to help persons with psychiatric illness to restore and rehabilitate functioning, to improve health and well-being, and to develop, maintain and express their most independent leisure lifestyle. During this year the staff of the Department of Recreation Therapy again functioned as active members of their respective interdisciplinary treatment teams. Their responsibilities included assessing patients' progress, participating in team meetings, maintaining their own level of professional preparedness, and contributing to the education and training of the many volunteers, students, new practitioners and interns that come to the Institute. The major focus of these treatment modalities was activity groups, but individual attention, in the form of educational, vocational and leisure counseling was also provided.

DEFINITION

It is a planned therapeutic activity aimed at enabling people with limitations to engage in recreational experiences.

AIMS OF RECREATIONAL THERAPY

- To encourage social interaction
- To decrease withdrawal tendencies
- To provide outlet for feeling
- To promote socially acceptable behavior
- To develop skills, talents and abilities
- To increase physical confidence and a feeling of self-worth.

POINTS TO BE KEPT IN MIND

1. Provide a nonthreatening and nondemanding environment.

2. Provide activities that are relaxing and without rigid guidelines and time frames.
3. Provide activities that are enjoyable and self-satisfying.

TYPES OF RECREATIONAL ACTIVITIES

a. *Motor forms*: These can be further divided into fundamental and accessory; among the fundamental forms are such games as hockey and football, while the accessory forms are exemplified by play activity and dancing.
b. *Sensory forms*: These can be either visual, e.g. looking at motion pictures, play, etc. or auditory such as listening to a concert.
c. *Intellectual forms*: These include reading debating and so on.

SUGGESTED RECREATIONAL ACTIVITIES FOR PSYCHIATRIC DISORDERS

a. *Anxiety disorders*: Aerobic activities like walking, jogging, etc.
b. *Depressive disorders*: Noncompetitive sports which provide outlet for anger like walking, jogging, running, etc.
c. *Manic disorders*: One-to-one basis individual game like badminton, ball.
d. *Schizophrenia*: (Paranoid) concentrative activities like chess, puzzles.
e. *Dementia*: Concrete, repetition crafts and projects that breed familiarization and comfort.
f. *Childhood and adolescence disorders*: It is better to work the child on a one-to-one basis and give him a feeling of importance. Some activities include playing, story telling, and painting.

Adolescences far better in groups; provide gross motor activities like sports and games to use up the excess energy.

g. *Mental retardation*: Activities should be according to the client's level of functioning such as walking, dancing, swimming, ball playing, etc.

ROLE OF NURSES IN RECREATIONAL THERAPY

1. Nurse must encourage the patient to communicate and express his feelings.
2. Nurse must provide a nonthreatening and nondemanding environment.
3. She must provide activities that are relaxing and without rigid guidelines.
4. She must provide activities that are enjoyable and self-satisfying.
5. Nurse must help patient to develop skill, talents abilities.
6. She must frequently observe clients behavior throughout the activities.
7. Nurse must promote socially acceptable behavior in the client.
8. The nurse must help the client to discuss specific situations in the life that produce the most distress and describe his or her response towards these situations.

Chapter 21 Relaxation Therapy

OVERVIEW

Stress is a part of life. It can be positive or negative but it can be eliminated keeping stress at a manageable level is a lifelong process. Relaxation therapy is an effective means of reducing the stress response in some individuals. The degree of anxiety that an individual experiences in response to stress is related to certain predisposing factors, such as characteristics of temperament with which he or she was born, past experiences resulting in learned patterns of responding and existing conditions such as health status, coping strategies and adequate support system. Various methods of relaxation therapy are presented.

DEEP BREATHING EXERCISES

Relaxation is accomplished by allowing the lungs to breathe in as much oxygen as possible. Air is breath slowly through the nose, held for a few seconds, and then exhaled slowly through the mouth. Breathing exercises have been found to be effective in reducing anxiety, depression, irritability, muscular tension and fatigue. An advantage of this type of exercise is that it can be accomplished anywhere at any time.

PROGRESSIVE RELAXATION TECHNIQUE

Each muscle group is tensed for 5–7 seconds and then relaxed for 20–30 seconds during which time the individual concentrates on the difference in sensation between two conditions. excellent result have been observed with this method in the treatment of muscular tension, anxiety, insomnia, depression, fatigue, muscle spasm, neck and back pain, high blood pressure, etc.

MODIFIED PROGRESSIVE MUSCLE RELAXATION TECHNIQUE OR PASSIVE MUSCLE RELAXATION TECHNIQUE

Relaxation is achieved with this method by passively concentrating on the feeling of relaxation within the muscle groups.

MEDITATION

The goal of meditation is to gain 'mastery over attention'. The basic component of meditation includes a quiet environment, a passive attitude, a comfortable position and a word or scene to focus on. It has been used successfully in the treatment of cardiovascular diseases, obsessive thinking, anxiety, and depression.

MENTAL IMAGERY

This method of relaxation employs the imagination in an effort to reduce the body's response to stress. The individual follows his/her imagination in selecting and environment considered to be relaxing, and concentrates on this relaxing image in an effort to achieve relaxation. Some might select a scene at the seashore, a mountain atmosphere or floating through the air in a white fluffy cloud. Soft background enhances the effect.

BIOFEEDBACK

Biofeedback uses a machine to reduce anxiety and modify behavioral responses. Small electrodes connected to the biofeedback equipment are attached to the patient's forehead. Brainwaves, muscle tension, body temperature, heart rate and blood pressure can be monitored for small changes. These change are communicated to the patient by auditory and visual means. Patients are more relaxed and patient become, the more pleasant are the sound and sights presented. These pleasant sights and sounds stops when the patient stops relaxing and they resume when the patient reaches the relaxed stage. It has been used successfully in treating hypertension, migraine headaches, muscle spasms/pain, anxiety, phobias, stuttering, and teeth grinding.

PHYSICAL EXERCISES

Physical exertion provides a natural outlet for the tension produced by the body. Following exercises, physiological equilibrium is restored resulting in as feeling of relaxation and revitalization. It helps in strengthening cardiovascular system, prevent obesity, relieve muscular tension, prevent muscle spasms, and reduce anxiety and depressions.

Chapter 22 Educational Therapy

INTRODUCTION

It is used when the client has problems of misconception. The educational therapist provides reading and learning experiences that can do a great deal to eliminate his misconceptions and anxiety.

This is a report of the use to which 'educational therapy' has been put at the Menninger Clinic. The author describes the classroom arrangement and the planning of the curriculum. As in other activities at the Clinic, special emphasis is placed on the individual needs of the patient. In addition to classroom facilities which are made available, the director of the program takes advantage of the educational facilities outside the Clinic. The need for close co-operation between the teacher and the patient's physician, as well as with directors of other activities, is emphasized.

EDUCATIONAL APPROACH

This description of an educational approach for adult psychiatric patients with childhood neuropsychiatric disorders can be seen as a general survey of how educational methods can be used in this context (Fig. 22.1).

It was not until the late1990s that the group of disorders described as being childhood neuropsychiatric in nature began to be regarded as a concern for adult psychiatry. That patients did not 'outgrow' these conditions but had symptoms to a greater or lesser extent into adulthood has become increasingly apparent. It has also been shown that the associated difficulties can actually worsen overtime as the demands for personal independence and responsibility-taking increase. Behaviors that could be accepted or excused in childhood become obvious problems in the adult. This can result in social exclusion, difficulties in managing independent living, work, home and relationships. The increased demands on a person with a low stress threshold can be so great that they result in a state of confusion and even psychosis. For some, the pressures of an incomprehensible world can lead to impulsive actions, violence and crime, which in turn lead to forensic psychiatric care (Siponmaa, Kristiansson, Gillberg, 1999).

A case study was presented: A woman, now 45-year-old, who has been treated for 30 years in adult psychiatry under different diagnoses was regarded as an extremely difficult and puzzling patient before she was diagnosed with autism.

Even if we are now becoming better at recognizing and diagnosing autism spectrum disorders in adults, there is no treatment method in adult psychiatry that is designed specifically for this group. A psychiatric diagnosis does not automatically stipulate the type of treatment that is needed. The intervention methods that until now have proven to be effective in dealing with autism are those based on an educational approach.

My own experiences from working in special education with adults who have autism spectrum disorders and are treated in adult psychiatric settings is the basis for the testing of an educational concept. It has been tested as a part of a further education for the staff in eight psychiatric units in three regions of Sweden. Six of the clinics have inpatients. Five of them have forensic psychiatric patients. The results will be presented in a doctoral thesis "*From Medication to Education. Persons with Autism in Adult Psychiatry*"(Mandre, 2002). It is based on an **Educational Diagnosis (Fig. 22.1)** that is derived from observations in the areas of:

- Perception/reactions
- Sensory modality
- Memory/thinking/verbal communication
- Contact/nonverbal communication
- Motor behavior.

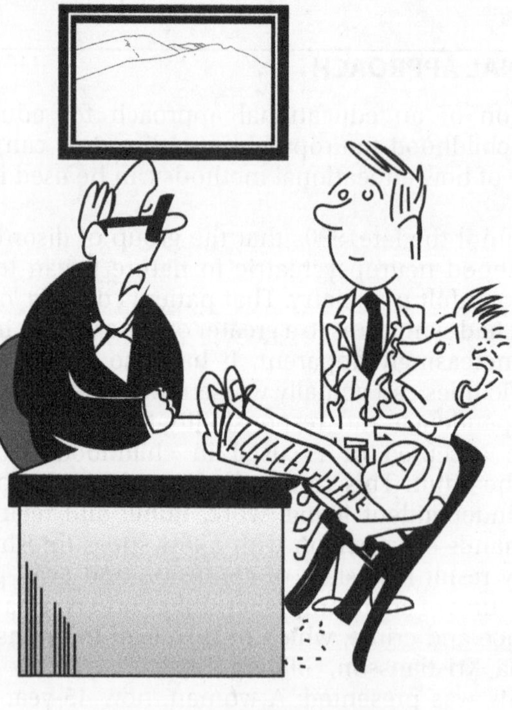

Figure 22.1: Educational diagnosis

EDUCATIONAL DIAGNOSIS

Perception/Reactions

It is common that people with autism have disturbances in perception and with sensory modulation, which are important to assess. Difficulties in making eye contact or over sensitivity to light may be sometimes be misinterpreted as paranoid reactions. A person who always puts his arms up in front of his face when he meets others can give the impression that he is afraid of radiation or other kinds of influence from people, while in reality he can have developed a strategy for avoiding eye contact and then made the gesture into a compulsive ritual.

People who are tactilely defensive do not willingly sit with others and usually try to be first or last in a queue to avoid contact. There are also people who absolutely cannot tolerate being touched by others, especially if it comes unexpectedly. A friendly hand on the shoulder can trigger a reflexive action such as kicking or punching. If others are not aware that these kinds of perceptual distortions exist, they may think the inappropriate behaviors are voluntary and an expression of aggressiveness.

Reactions to one's surroundings and the speed at which a person moves from impulse to action are also crucial in devising educational strategies and deciding which methods can be used. They have to be completely different for a person with immediate, reflexive reactions than for someone who has delayed reactions that require extra time to process.

Sensory Modality

Information comes into our consciousness through our senses—Auditorily, visually or tacitly (Fig. 22.2). The sensory channel through which we learn best and remember information is not always the auditory, by means of spoken language. If the person in question has short-term memory problems, he or she needs to find ways of storing information so that all of its parts are accessible for processing thought and solving problems. This means that people who have memory difficulties also need memory aids. Printed and accessible daily schedules are examples of such.

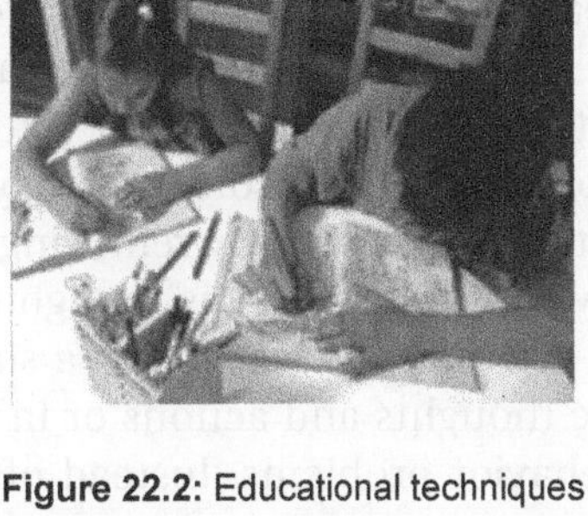

Figure 22.2: Educational techniques

In the case of autism spectrum disorders, common educational advice is that there always should be visual schedules and clarifications. There are exceptions to this rule. One group, which could be called a subtype in the autism spectrum, is described as having NLD (Nonverbal Learning Disabilities or right-hemisphere dysfunction) and requires a different kind of treatment, in that these people are dependent on auditory information. Since they are very verbal, it is easy to overestimate their ability to understand language. They can have an extensive vocabulary and spout forth borrowed expression that they do not understand at all, just as they find it hard to understand what others mean. When you know that these difficulties exist, you can get in the habit of asking for a clarification to be sure of how much of what has been said has been understood. You may have to reformulate and simplify your language a number of times before these patients know what is actually meant. Their way of processing information is based on details and they can get stuck on them in a round about way and go over them again and again without being able to ever get to the point.

Memory/Thinking/Verbal Communication

Memory problems and perceptual disturbances affect a person's interpretation and experience of the world. This means that thinking and verbal communication are also affected by the person's distorted interpretation of the world. If he has a concrete vocabulary in which everything is taken literally, and has difficulties to perceive unspoken messages, he can end up having repeated confrontations with his surroundings.

- **Example**: A young man with several childhood neuropsychiatric diagnoses has become a troublesome patient on a unit for patients requiring a high level of care. Staff member report that he is aggressive and hits and they end up putting him in isolation, where he destroys everything in the room. They phase out all regular contact and all forms of activities during his first weeks on the unit. A large number of people take turns guarding him. A sense of hopelessness spreads through the unit, where the staff feel that they have done all they can and only want to send him some place elsewhere they know how to 'deal' with these conditions. The young man's own explanation for the violence can be that the staff have 'cleared their throats too much' or used words that he misunderstood. Most likely these words were meant as a good-natured attempt to make contact or as a joke that the patient did not get. Staff members probably could have dealt constructively with the violence by not punishing the patient right away by removing everything that gave him something with which to occupy his thoughts. By prohibiting him from participating in activities, he was left in a sort of mental vacuum filled with compulsive thoughts and actions or in total passivity, which only increased his behavior problems. Instead of seeing an individual with perceptual disturbances with a distorted and very concrete way of thinking for whom special adjustments had to be made by those who interacted with him, all the blame was placed on him, as if he had consciously decided to act out and could have refrained from doing so by making an effort at self-control. With such an interpretation of the problem, the situation had become a catch-22, impossible to get out of (Fig. 22.3).

It is usually said the people with high functioning autism have a large memory capacity. They can also have an exceptional ability to learn facts by heart and to behave like little professors in astronomy at a young age or be specialists on antelopes of Africa or maps of the world. By remembering details or collecting factual information, they stand out as though they had a 'good memory'. Demands greater than they can handle are often expected of them in other areas where their memory skills are considerably poorer. It can be much more difficult for them to place the details in the bigger picture and understand them in context. Remembering facts that can be repeated does not mean that one really has knowledge in the subject area. To have knowledge means that one is able to transform the information to new knowledge that can be generalized to other, similar situations. If we are impressed by the 'good' memory of these patients, we can be totally mislead. It is more productive to examine which functions of memory work well which work poorly.

***Endel Tulving's theoretical memory model divides memory functions as follows*:**

- Procedural memory, which is noncognitive. This is where we store motor actions, conditioned behaviors and simple associative chains of action.

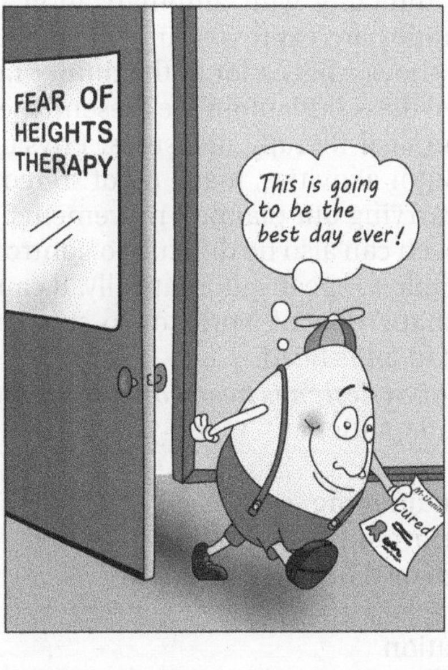
FEAR OF
HEIGHTS
THERAPY
This is going to be the best day ever!
Cured

Figure 22.3: Educational therapy for anxiety

- Perceptual memory, which stores shapes and structures such as the visual and auditory shapes of words. This memory enables us to categorize objects according to different characteristics.
- Semantic memory, which is cognitive and stores factual information.
- Episodic memory, which stores episodes that have been personally experienced. Poor episodic memory results in a fragmented self-image.
- Short-term memory, which stores information for a short time in order to interpret and compare it to other material in one's memory. Important for problem solution.

Contact/Nonverbal Communication

When people with autism spectrum disorders are treated in psychiatric care, they encounter many assumptions that are taken for granted as to what they are supposed to know and understand about social situations and of how to communicate with people in their environment.

Human contact presupposes an innate ability to 'read' other people. Those who process information in great detail can have difficulties putting all the details together to make a whole, and so are unable to get a general impression of others. They find it difficult to interpret other's feelings in social situations. In all social interaction there is a rhythm; an inability in getting a feel for and following this rhythm produces a sense that something is wrong in social situations.

Motor Behavior

All automatic movements are types of motor activity. Some people have considerably more difficulty with automatization than others. Motor coordination difficulties are expressed in clumsiness; the person has a hard time tying his shoes, spills a lot at the dinner table and has sloppy table manners. When these difficulties are present, there is a need for both educational and physical therapy measures. Physical restlessness and hyperactivity are motor activities, made up of stereotypical movements and difficulties in carrying out planned movements. The motor activity of the organs of speech can also be difficult to control. This means that a person may not be able to speak automatically. It can be hard to express oneself in an automatic flow of words or to speak words that are not already thought out in one's head.

Individual educational design is based on a combination of—

- Environmental adaptations
- Structure
- Habituation/conditioning
- Whole concept learning
- Learning through own insight
- Social learning
- Fantasy, imagination
- Educational content.

Environmental adaptations for—

- Disruptions in perception
- High degree of impulsivity
- Destructive behavior.

Environmental adaptations can involve—

- Sound absorption measures
- Sparse furnishings and interior decoration
- Built-in, clearly defined limits
- Well-defined areas of activity, so that it is clear what is to be done where
- People to set limits when internalized limitations are lacking.

A structure that—

- Offers security, predictability
- Provides an overview
- It is a support for learning (but has no value of its own and should be modified or removed when its purpose is fulfilled).

Habituation/conditioning as learning method—

- When impulsivity/destructiveness are present
- When a high level of compulsiveness exists which is bothersome to those in the surroundings but not to the person himself
- When the person lacks insight into his problems.

This method teaches a person to do something in a certain manner. No personal insight or reflection about the learning is needed. Automatization of actions or series of actions.

Whole concept learning—

- When the person lacks metacognition ('I know what I know and what I am capable of').
- When the person is capable of learning things by rote.
- When the person needs to learn patterns, as in social situations.

A person can learn something when it is related to a given situation or context. This is rote learning without personal reflection and the knowledge thus gained cannot be lifted out of that context and generalized to others.

Learning through own insight—

- Requires metacognition.

When a person has the ability to think about his own thought processes and is aware of what he knows and what he does not know, he can learn by gaining greater and greater understanding. His way of thinking and his actions are altered by new knowledge. What is known can be lifted out from its original context and applied in comparable situations. When a person has reached this level of thinking and metacognition, cognitive therapy can be an alternative form of treatment.

Social learning—

Patients who are unable to intuitively 'read' social situations are in need of tools to help them better cope.

Learning in a social context, for example, in a social group whose purpose is to teach social behavior.

Fantasy, imagination as a learning method—

- For establishing contact
- To think through alternative scenarios and their consequences
- To increase flexibility of thought.

Educational content—

- Practical daily-living skills
- Knowledge of people, social rules
- Second-hand knowledge that can be found in books and from the experiences of others in order to learn new things, gain information and for intellectual stimulation.

Chapter 23

Bibliotherapy

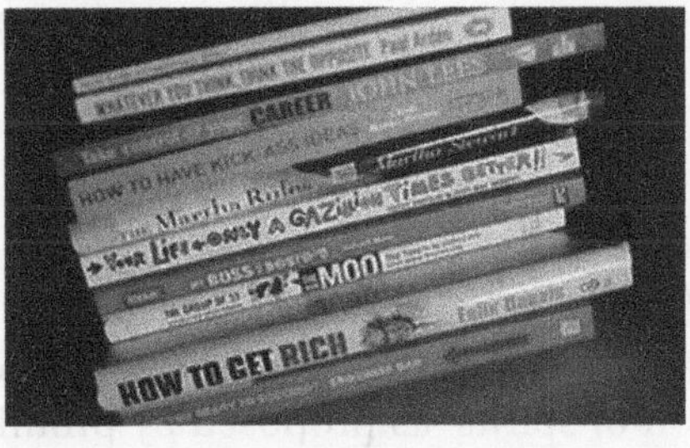

Figure 23.1: Bibliographies

INTRODUCTION

It is described as the prescription of reading materials (Fig. 23.1) that will help to develop emotional maturity and sustain mental health.

RESEARCH ABSTRACT

The guided use of selected books as an adjunct to treatment is applicable to patients in all stages of life and with a variety of problems. This paper describes the authors' experience using books as an adjunct to therapy with psychiatric patients. The authors define the term, review the literature, and set out the objectives of bibliotherapy. The paper presents some principles to follow when assigning books and examples of books used for common problems. Finally, examples are given of bibliotherapy in action at two Ontario Hospitals, and some future directions are suggested.

BIBLIOTHERAPY: PATIENT LIBRARIES AND READING PROGRAMS, ONE COMPONENT OF THE MORAL TREATMENT REVOLUTION

Abstract

Objectives

We will examine the utilization of bibliotherapy in 19th century psychiatric 'asylums' focusing on two respected institutions; Butler Hospital and Worcester State Hospital as well as the writings of their respective superintendents, Isaac Ray MD and Samuel B Woodward MD METHODS: Merriam-Webster's Dictionary defines bibliotherapy as 'the use of reading materials for help in solving personal problems or for psychiatric therapy'. 'Bibliotherapy' first appears in the literature in conjunction with the work of Anna Freud in the early 20th century. However, it was being used extensively within the practice of the 'moral therapy' movement in mental health institutions in the 1800's. In the many new American public and private psychiatric hospitals that were being founded at that time, superintendent/physicians saw reading as one of many 'occupational therapies' that would assist in the recovery of the institutionalized patient. We will examine primary resources describing patient library services, focusing specifically on the works of Woodward, Ray and others of the thirteen 'revolutionary' founders of the group which eventually became the American Psychiatric Association and which held its first meeting in Philadelphia in 1844 (Fig. 23.2).

Results and conclusions

Were 'cheap novels' a cause of insanity (as Ray wrote) or a diversion from the 'depression of spirits' as proposed by prominent Philadelphia physician Benjamin Rush (1745–1813)? Would newspapers 'help' patients stay current or would they or 'hurt' by exposing them to horrors of life outside? These were some of the questions being asked by leaders of America's early psychiatric institutions. Nonetheless, bibliotherapy was a foundational treatment of the moral therapy era and it appears that most if not all new institutions of the time had therapeutic reading programs and/or patient libraries. While neither Woodward nor Ray wrote extensively on this subject in their Annual Reports or correspondence, there is ample evidence in the primary literature of the importance of bibliotherapy. We will demonstrate this through the use of quotations, images, sketches and examples of items on the shelves of patient libraries in the early to mid 1800's.

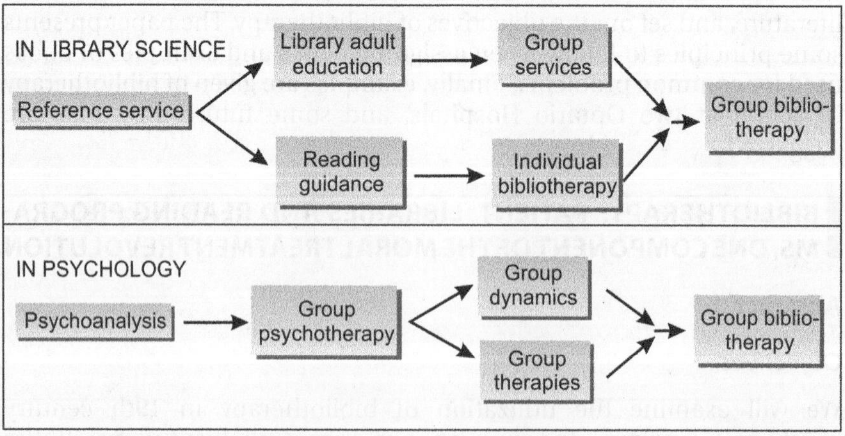

Figure. 23.2: Bibliotherapy in psychology

Chapter 24 Play Therapy

INTRODUCTION

Play is a natural mode of growth and development in children. Through play a child learns to express his emotions and it serves as a tool in the development of the child.

CURATIVE FUNCTIONS

1. It releases tension and pent up emotions.
2. It allows compensation for loss and failures.
3. It improves emotional growth through his relationship with other children.
4. It provides an opportunity to the child to act out his fantasies and conflicts to get rid of aggression and to learn positive qualities from other children.

DIAGNOSTIC FUNCTIONS

1. Play therapy gives the therapist a chance to explore family relationships of the child and discover what difficulties are contributing to the child's problems.
2. Play therapy allows to study hidden aspects of the child's personality.
3. It is possible to obtain a good idea of the intelligence level of the child.
4. Through play intersibling relationships can be adequately studied.

TYPES OF PLAY THERAPY

a. **Individual vs group play therapy**: In individual therapy the child is allowed to play by himself and the therapist's attention is focused on this one child alone.
   In group therapy other children are involved.
b. **Free play vs controlled play therapy**: In free play the child is given freedom in deciding with what toys he wants to play.
   In controlled play therapy the child is introduced into a scene where the situation or setting is already established.
c. **Structured vs unstructured play therapy**: Structured play therapy involves organizing the situation in such a way so as to obtain more information.

In unstructured play therapy no situation is set and no plans are followed.

d. **Directive vs nondirective play therapy**: In Directive play therapy the therapist totally sets the directions whereas in nondirective play therapy the child receives no directions.

ROLE OF NURSE IN PLAY THERAPY

1. The nurse must select the type of play that the child must indulge into.
2. The nurse through her observations of the client's behavior during the play activity will gain valuable information that she can subsequently utilize to therapeutic advantages in the client treatment.
3. She must provide for a nonthreatening and nondemanding environment.
4. She must provide games that are enjoyable.
5. Through play therapy she can explore family relationships of the child and discover what difficulties are contributing to child's problems.

Chapter 25 Music Therapy

INTRODUCTION

Music therapy is the functional application of music towards the attainment of specific therapeutic goals.

Music can be beneficial for anyone. Although it can be used therapeutically for people who have physical, emotional, social or cognitive deficits, even those who are healthy can use music to relax, reduce stress, improve mood, or to accompany exercise. There are no potentially harmful or toxic effects. Music therapist help their patients achieve a number of goals through music, including improving movement of communication, academic strengths, attention span, motor skills they may also assist with behavioral therapy and pain management.

DEFINITION

'Music therapy is defined as the use of music in accomplishment of therapeutic aims'.

The restoration, maintenance, improvement of mental health and physical health.

The music may be recorded music, song writing movement and music instruments.

According to Alvin (1975), 'defines music therapy as the controlled use of music in the treatment, education, training and rehabilitation of children and adult suffering from physical, mental, or emotional disorders'.

According to Brusica (1930), describe music therapy is an interpersonal process in which therapist in all of its facets—Physical, emotional, mental, social, esthetic and spiritual-helps client to improve or maintain a state of health. He observes further that music therapy is a systematic process of intervention wherein the therapist helps the client to achieve health, using musical experiences and help the relationships that develop through them as a dynamic force of change.

According to Mereni (2004), indicates that the word therapy comes from the Greek word 'therapeia' which means 'healing' in the same sense as treatment of a disease.

'A curative intervention for the purpose of healing a sickness or restoring health'. Music therapy has to do with musical intervention.

Mereni however remarks that music therapy is not listening to music for relaxation, to relieve boredom, and/or to relieve pain or physical aches, or to listen to music to induce sleep. In his view such instances offer proof of the power of music and such a power can then be involved when we set out to employ music as the tool of therapeutic intervention. In the most cases in Nigeria, music and dance are closely knit.

GOALS

The goals of music therapy are dependent upon the purpose of music therapy for each individual case. Drug and alcohol centers and schools may use music therapy and behavior changing may be an important goal. Whereas, nursing homes may use music therapy in more of a support role or to relieve pain. Some of the goals of music therapy may include:

- It increases communication skills.
- It helps in expression of feelings (aggressive feeling by loudly singing in the group singing in the group song).
- Improve self-esteem.
- Reduces maladaptive (stereotype, compulsive, self-abusive), etc.
- Improve fine and gross motor skills, auditory perception.
- Helping the patient take their focus away from their grief or pain.
- Altering the patient behavior.
- Improving the patient's social skills.
- Allowing the patient to think creatively and develop their imagination.
- Helping the patient deal with a rehabilitative process.

TYPES OF MUSIC THERAPY

There are different types of music therapy that are used according to the patient's needs although music therapy should not be labeled, as each patient is different and should be assessed on an individual basis, understanding some of the different uses of music therapy, types of music therapy can help as appreciate the different uses of music therapy. Music therapies' activities can be loosely divided into the following categories:

- Music therapy to help develop communication, language, and intellectual development.
- Music therapy as support, for people who are grieving, going through a crisis time or who are in pain.
- Music therapy is to lowers stress and tension.
- Music therapy as a motivation for rehabilitation.
- Music therapy is to encourage movement.
- Music therapy as a means to identify with cultural and spiritual identity.
- Music therapy to assist memory and imagination.

PURPOSES OF MUSIC THERAPY

Physical Effects

- Brain function physically changes in response to music.
- The rhythm can guide the body into breathing in slower, deeper patterns that have a calming effect.
- Heart rate and blood pressure are always responsive to the types of music that are listened to. The speed of heartbeat tends to speed or slow depending on the volume and speed of the auditory stimulus.
- Louder and faster notices tend to raise both heart rate and blood pressure; slower, softer, more regular tones produce the opposite result.
- Music can also relieve muscle tension and improve motor skills. It is often used to help rebuild physical parenting skills in rehabilitation clinics.
- Levels of endorphins, natural pain relieves, are increased while listening to music, and levels of stress hormones are decreased.
- This latter effect may partially explain the ability of music to improve immune function. A 1993 study at Michigan state university showed that even 15 minutes of exposure to music could increase interleukin levels, a consequence which also heightens immunity.

Mental Effects

- Depending upon the type and style of sound, music can either sharpen mental acuity or assist in relaxation.
- Memory and learning can be enhanced, and this is used with good results in children with learning disabilities.
- This effects may also be partially due to increased concentration that many people have while listening to music. Better productivity is another outcome of an improved ability to concrete.
- The term 'Mozart effect' was coined after a study showed that college students performed better on math problems when listening to classical music.

Emotional Effects

- The ability of music to influence human emotion is well known, and is used extensively by movie makers.
- A variety of musical moods may be used to create feelings of calmness, tension, excitement, or romance.
- Lullabies have long been popular for soothing babies to sleep, music also be used to express emotions nonverbally, which can be a very valuable therapeutic tool in some settings.

ADVANTAGES

1. Facilitate emotional expressions.
2. Improve cognitive skills like—learning and listening skills.

3. Exercises through body movements.
4. Maintain muscle tone.
5. Social interaction is stimulated.

GUIDELINES FOR EFFECTIVE MUSIC THERAPY

The following guidelines to maximize the effectiveness of the music therapy—

- To wash away stress, try taking a 20 minute 'sound bath'.
- Put some relaxing music on your stereo, then lie in a comfortable position on a couch or on the floor near the speakers.
- For a deeper experience, you can wear headphones to focus your attention and to avoid distraction.
- Choose music with a slow rhythm. Slower than the natural heartbeat. Music that a repeating or cyclical pattern is found to be effective in most people.
- As the music plays, allow it to wash over you, rising of the stress from the day. Focus on your breathing letting it deepen, slow and become regular.
- Concentrate on the silence between the notes in the music; this keeps you from analyzing the music and makes relaxation more complete.
- If you need stimulation after a day of work, go for a faster music rather than slow calming music.
- When going gets tough, go for music, you are familiar with such a childhood favorite and favorite oldies. Familiarity often breeds calmness.
- Take walks with your favorite music playing on the walkman. Inhale and exhale in tune with the music.
- Listening the sounds of nature, such as ocean waves or the calm of a deep forest, can reduce stress. Try taking 15–20 minute walk if you are near the seashore or a quite patch of woods.

ASPECTS OF MUSIC THERAPY

Mereni (1997) identified some healing aspects of music/dance as restorative agents and they are—

1. Anxiolytic music therapy— Aims to free one from fear, fright or anxiety.
2. Tensionlytic music therapy— Aims to relieve one from physical and mental tension resulting from manual and spiritual labor.
3. Algolytic music therapy— Aims to relieve physical pain.
4. Psycholytic music therapy— Aims to loosen a person from the group of evil spirits.
5. Patholytic music therapy— Aims to relieve the grief of bereavement.

HOW DOES THE MUSIC THERAPY WORKS?

Music therapy works in conjunction with a therapist. The music therapist will assess the emotional and physical health of the patient through musical responses and then design music sessions based on the client's needs. Music therapy works in a number of different ways as music helps the patient do different things and provides different benefits. Some of the ways that music therapy may help patients include:

- By keeping the patient's attention
- By structuring time
- By providing an enjoyable method of repetition
- By helping memory
- By encouraging movements
- By tapping into memories and emotions.

WHERE DO MUSIC THERAPIST WORKS?

Music therapist works in a variety of different places. Some of those places include;

- Psychiatric hospital, working with the mentally ill
- Medical hospitals, working with all type of patients
- Rehabilitative facilities
- Day care treatment centers
- Community mental centers
- Drug and alcohol programs
- Nursing homes and senior centers, working with music therapy and the elderly correctional facilities
- Schools.

NURSES' ROLE IN MUSIC THERAPY

1. Organizing music program for the patient by the patient
2. Encourage patient to participate in music activities
3. Observe their nonverbal expression during music
4. Provide positive reward to participation in the program.

RESEARCH REVIEW

Music Therapy and Depression

Music therapy may help some patients to fight against depression, according to review published in 2008. Researches sized up data from five previously published studies, four of which found that participants receiving music therapy were more likely to see a decrease in depression symptoms (compared to those who did not receive music therapy). According to the review's authors, patients appeared to experience the greatest benefits when therapists used theory-based therapeutic techniques, such as, painting to music and improvized singing.

Chapter 26

Dance Therapy

INTRODUCTION

It is a psychotherapeutic use of movement, which furthers the emotional and physical integration of the individuals.

ADVANTAGES

1. Helps to develop body awareness.
2. Facilitates expression of feelings.
3. Improve interaction and communication.
4. Foster integration of physical, emotional, and social experiences that increase sense of self-confidence.

Dance therapy, or **dance movement therapy** is the *psychotherapeutic* use of movement and *dance* for emotional, *cognitive, social, behavioral,* and *physical* conditions. As a form of *expressive therapy,* DMT is founded on the basis that movement and emotion are directly related. The ultimate purpose of DMT is to find a healthy balance and sense of wholeness (Fig. 26.1).

Since its birth in the 1940s, DMT has gained much popularity and has been taken to more serious and beneficial levels. Over the years, the practices of DMT have progressed; however, the main principles that founded this form of therapy have remained the same. Influenced by the 'main principles' of this therapy, most DMT sessions are configured

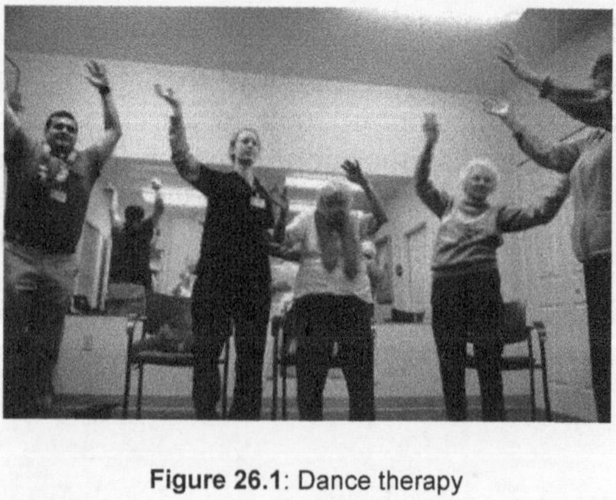

Figure 26.1: Dance therapy

around four main stages: Preparation, incubation, illumination, and evaluation. Organizations such as the *American Dance Therapy Association* and the Association for Dance Movement Therapy, United Kingdom maintain the high standards of profession and education throughout the field. DMT is practiced in places such as mental health rehabilitation centers, medical and educational settings, nursing homes, day care facilities, and other health promotion programs. This form of therapy which is taught in a wide array of locations goes farther than just centering the body. Specialized treatments of DMT can help cure and aid many types of diseases and disabilities. Other common names for DMT include: Movement psychotherapy and dance therapy.

HISTORY

Although dance has been a method of expression for centuries, it wasn't until just recently that it was characterized as a form of therapy. The development of DMT can be split into two waves throughout history. Long before the first wave of DMT in *America* (1940s), the *UK* developed the idea of dance therapy. The first records of dance being used as a form of therapy date as far back as the nineteenth century in the *UK*. Although there were significant *American* influences, the main theories of dance therapy originated in the *UK* (Fig. 26.2).

First Wave

Marian Chace, 'The Grand Dame' of dance therapy, is the woman responsible for introducing the idea of DMT to the *United States* and therefore inspiring the first wave of DMT. She is considered the principal founder of what is now dance therapy in the *United States*. In 1942, through her work, dance was first introduced to western *medicine*. Chace was originally a *dancer*, *choreographer*, and performer. After opening her own *dance* school in *Washington, DC*, Chace began to realize the effects of dance and movement had on her students. She was soon asked to

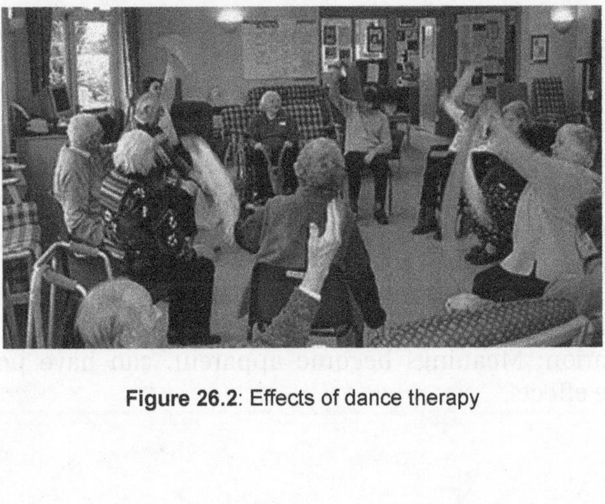

Figure 26.2: Effects of dance therapy

work at *St. Elizabeth's Hospital* in *Washington, DC* once psychiatrists too realized the benefits their patients were receiving from attending Chace's dance classes. In 1966, Chace became the First President of the *American Dance Therapy Association*, an organization which she and several other DMT pioneers founded.

Second Wave

It wasn't until the *1970s* and *80s* that the second wave of DMT came around and sparked much interest from American therapists. During this time, therapists began to experiment with the psychotherapeutic applications of *dance* and movement. As a result of the therapists experiments, DMT was then categorized as a form of *psychotherapy*. It was from this second wave that today's DMT evolved.

PRINCIPLES

The theory of DMT is based upon the idea that 'the body and mind are inseparable'.

'Dance movement therapy rests on certain theoretical principles. These are:

- *Body* and *mind* interact, so that a change in movement will affect total functioning.
- Movement reflects personality.
- The therapeutic relationship is mediated at least to some extent nonverbally, for example through the therapist mirroring the client's movement.
- Movement contains a symbolic function and as such can be evidence of *unconscious* process.
- Movement *improvization* allows the client to experiment with new ways of being.
- DMT allows for the recapitulation of early object relationships by virtue of the largely nonverbal mediation of the latter'.

Through the unity of the *body, mind,* and *spirit,* DMT provides a sense of wholeness to all individuals.

THE CREATIVE PROCESS

The creative process has four stages, which occur during DMT. Each stage contains a smaller set of goals which correlate to the larger purpose of DMT. The stages and goals of DMT vary with each individual. Although the stages are progressive, the stages are usually revisited several times throughout the entire DMT process. The four stages are:

- Preparation: The warm-up stage, safety is established.
- Incubation: Relaxed, let go of conscious control, movements become symbolic.
- Illumination: Meanings become apparent, can have positive and negative effects.

- Evaluation: Discuss significance of the process, prepare to end therapy.

SPECIALIZED TREATMENTS

DMT can be used to heal serious disorders and *diseases*. Although DMT is promoted to reduce *stress* and center the body, this therapy is very effective in helping to heal other disabilities and *diseases*. Examples of these include:

- *Autism*: Therapists connect on a sensory-motor level, provides a sense of acceptance and expands skills and cognitive abilities, increases maturity.
- *Learning disabilities*: Develops better organizational skills, learns/experiences control and choice, higher self-confidence, new inspirations to learn.
- *Mental retardation*: Improves body image, social skills, coordination, and motor skills, promotes communication.
- *Deaf and hearing impaired*: It reduces feelings of isolation, provides inspiration for relationships.
- *Blind and visually impaired*: It improves body image, motor skills, and personal awareness.
- *Physically handicapped*: It improves motor skills and body image, provides a way to communicate and express emotions.
- *Elderly*: It provides social interaction, expression, and exercise, alleviates fears of loneliness and isolation.
- *Eating disorders*: It alters distorted body images which helps end destructive behaviors, discovers symbolic meanings behind disorder/food.
- *PTSD*: It weaves together past and present through symbolism in a 'safe place' to confront painful memories.
- *Parkinson's disease*: It uses rhythm to help reduce body dysfunctions which improves motor abilities, balance, and use of limbs.
- *Holistic birth preparation*: It implores relaxation techniques to reduce anxiety, learn breathing techniques and release energy, builds confidence to help cope with labor, birth and early parenting.

LOCATIONS

DMT is practiced in a large variety of locations. Such locations include:

- Rehabilitation centers
- Medical settings
- Educational settings
- Forensic settings
- Nursing homes
- Day care facilities
- Disease prevention centers
- Health promotion program.

ORGANIZATIONS

Organizations such as the *American Dance Therapy Association* were created in order to uphold high standards in the field of DMT. Such organizations help to connect individuals to therapists and DMT.

American Dance Therapy Association

American Dance Therapy Association (ADTA) was founded in 1966 in order to uphold high standards throughout dance therapy. The *ADTA* was created by Marian Chace, the First President of the *ADTA*, and other pioneers in dance movement. Along with setting standards for which therapists must attain to become licensed therapists, *ADTA* keeps an updated registry of all movement/dance therapists who have met *ADTA's* standards. In addition, *ADTA* also publishes the American Journal of Dance Therapy and sponsors annual professional conferences.

Association for Dance Movement Therapy, United Kingdom

The Association for Dance Movement Therapy, United Kingdom (ADMTUK) was one of the first organizations established to regulate the field of dance therapy. ADMTUK accredits therapists and oversees that all regulations are followed.

THERAPIST QUALIFICATIONS

ADTA is the main regulator of the required education and training in order to become a dance/movement therapist. Typically, a *master's degree* is required to become a dance/movement therapist. 'Dance Therapist Registered (DTR)' is the title given to beginner-level dance therapists who have had a minimum 700 hours of clinical training. For those who have completed over 3,640 hours of clinical work, they hold the title 'Academy of Dance Therapists (ADTR)'.

Chapter 27 Art Therapy

The goal of the art therapy is to help the patient express his thoughts, emotions and feelings through the drawings.

IMPORTANCE

- It is used as a diagnostic and therapeutic purposes
- It provide socially acceptable outlet for fantasy and wish fulfillment
- It helps the patient to gain relief from anxiety by graphically representing conflict and aggressive and traumatic material without guilt.

HISTORY

Art— Over one hundred years ago, a number of European writers described the spontaneous art done by patients in mental hospitals. This seemingly irrepressible urge to make art out of any available materials confirms the compelling power of artistic expression to reveal inner experience. It was because art making provided a means of expression for those who were often uncommunicative that art therapy came to be developed as one of the helping professions.

Art therapy is defined as a human service profession that uses art media, images, the creative process, and patient/client responses to the created products as reflections of an individual's development, abilities, personality, interests, concerns, and conflicts. Art therapy practice is based on knowledge of human developmental and psychological theories which are implemented in the full spectrum of models of assessment and treatment including educational, psychodynamic, cognitive, transpersonal, and other therapeutic means of reconciling emotional conflicts, fostering self-awareness, developing social skills, managing behavior, solving problems, reducing anxiety, aiding reality orientation, and increasing self-esteem.

Art therapy as a separate field developed simultaneously in England and the United States. Margaret Naumburg is considered its founder in this country. An educator and psychotherapist who started the Walden School in New York City, Naumburg wrote several books on art therapy and its applications with psychiatric patients in the 1940s and 1950s. Her sister Florence Cane modified principles from art education for use with children. At the same time, artists (including some who were conscientious objectors during the World War II) were volunteers in mental hospitals. They eventually convinced psychiatrists of the contributions art therapy could make to treating the most difficult patients.

Theories from psychoanalysis and art education are the foundations for the two poles of the field which are termed art psychotherapy and art as therapy. Whether the therapeutic process is inherent in talking about a work of art and in expressing oneself or in the specific act of creation has been a subject of considerable debate. Most art therapists find that they draw from both approaches, modifying what they do or emphasize according to the population with which they are working.

The first journal in the field was published in 1961 as the Bulletin of Art Therapy (now the American Journal of Art Therapy). The American Art Therapy Association (AATA), founded in 1969, is the national professional organization; it sponsors annual conferences and regional symposia, approves training programs, and publishes the journal Art Therapy. The first graduate degrees were awarded in the 1970s. Today, there are undergraduate introductory courses and preparatory programs in colleges across the country as well as 27 master's programs approved by AATA.

Art therapy is an effective treatment for the developmentally, medically, educationally, socially, or psychologically impaired; and is practiced in mental health, rehabilitation, medical, educational, and forensic institutions. Populations of all ages, races, and ethnic backgrounds are served by art therapists in individual, couples, family and group therapy formats.

Educational, professional and ethical standards for art therapists are regulated by the American Art Therapy Association. The Art Therapy Credentials Board, an independent organization, grants postgraduate registration (ATR) after reviewing documentation of completion of graduate education and postgraduate supervised experience. The Registered Art Therapist who successfully completes the written examination administered by the Art Therapy Credentials Board is qualified as Board Certified (ATR-BC), a credential requiring maintenance through continuing education credits.

Research in art therapy has included studying the influence of depression on the content of drawings, the use of art to assess cognitive skills, the correlation of psychiatric diagnosis and formal variables in art, and the effect of art therapy interventions as measured by single-case designs.

Chapter 28 Light Therapy

In the early 1980's, scientists researching depression noted a **consistent pattern of symptoms becoming more severe in many patients during the long winter months**, particularly in the northern hemisphere. Significantly, these symptoms eased or disappeared completely as the longer summer days returned.

In 1982 The National Institute of Health *(NIH)* identified winter depression and coined the term, 'SAD' for *Seasonal Affective Disorder*.

The scientists found that 'SAD' was related to an imbalance in the body's *natural circadian rhythms*. The Circadian rhythm or the body's inner clock **governs the timing of sleep, hormone production, body temperature, and other biological functions**.

In 1984, these pioneering scientists discovered that **exposure to bright white light is very effective at treating seasonal affective disorder**.

For many years, doctors had relegated light therapy to the periphery of credible science. It wasn't until 2001 that researchers from NIH, Thomas Jefferson Medical University and Apollo Health fully **understood how exposure to specialized bright light, stimulates the production of brain chemicals** to relieve the symptoms associated with seasonal depression.

Dr George Brainard's team at Thomas Jefferson Medical University, identified a **photo receptor in the human eye**, responsible for reacting to light and controlling the production of *melatonin*.

They found **specifically that light in the range of 447–484 nm (nanometers) is responsible for suppressing melatonin production and shifting circadian rhythms**. Indeed, this particular bandwidth of light is upto ten times more effective than other wavelengths. We now know this technology as **BLUEWAVE**.

When the recipient is exposed to Apollo's **BLUEWAVE Technology**, waves of light enter the eye. A nerve that connects the retina to a key point in the hypothalamus region of the brain is activated. Once activated the hypothalamus sends a signal to the pineal gland. The pineal gland immediately suppresses the withdrawal hormone Melatonin and stimulates the production of the active hormone *Serotonin*.

As *Serotonin* is released you become **more active, energetic and alert**. This action **improves concentration and motivation**.

Light therapy is a way to treat seasonal affective disorder, depression and certain other conditions by exposure to bright artificial light. During light therapy, you sit or work near a device called a light therapy box. The light therapy box gives off bright light that mimics natural outdoor light. Exposure to bright light from a light therapy box is thought to alter your circadian rhythms and suppress your body's natural release of melatonin. Together, these cause biochemical changes in your brain that help reduce or control symptoms of seasonal affective disorder and other conditions. Light therapy is also known as bright light therapy or phototherapy.

ADVANTAGES

- The advantages of light therapy include the fact that it is rather noninvasive with relatively few and minor side effects.
- Additionally, a significant number of people respond very quickly to this treatment.

DISADVANTAGES

- The disadvantages of light therapy comprise the daily commitment of time and investment in the equipment.
- Some health care providers have the light boxes available in their offices, but this necessitates a daily visit to the doctor.
- There are companies that rent the equipment. However, insurance does not always cover the expenses associated with this type of treatment. Also, relapse of symptoms is usually quite rapid after cessation of treatment.

LIGHT THERAPY USED FOR

- Migraine headache
- PMS (premenstrual syndrome)
- Insomnia and other sleep disorders
- SAD (seasonal affective disorder)
- Coldsores
- ADD/ADHD (attention deficit disorder)
- Stress reduction and relaxation
- CFS (chronic fatigue) and ME
- Pain reduction and management
- Acne and other skin problems
- Wound healing
- Medical applications for light therapy.

HOW DOES LIGHT THERAPY WORKS?

- When the recipient is expose to Apollo's BLUEWAVE technology, waves of light enter the eye.
- A nerve that connects the retina to a key pointing the hypothalamus region of the brain is activated.

- Once activated the hypothalamus sends a signal to the pineal gland. The pineal gland immediately suppresses the withdrawal hormone Melatonin and stimulates the production of the active hormone Serotonin.
- The therapeutic level of illumination has several known physiological effects, though its therapeutic mechanism is still unclear.
- Blood levels of the light-sensitive hormone melatonin, which may be abnormally high at certain times of day, are rapidly reduced by light exposure.
- Depending on when bright light is presented, the bodies internal clock—which controls daily rhythms of body temperature, hormone secretion, and sleep patterns—shifts ahead or is delayed when stimulated by light.
- These physiological time shifts may be the basis of the therapeutic response.
- Light may also amplify the day-night difference in these rhythms. Research into the possible mechanisms is currently underway, and the final answer is not yet in.

HOW IS IT DELIVERED? (FIG. 28.1)

- Light therapy involves exposure to intense levels of light under controlled conditions.
- The recommended light therapy system consists of a set of fluorescent bulbs installed in a box with a diffusing screen, and set up on a table or desktop at which one can sit comfortably for the treatment session.
- Treatment consists simply of sitting close to the light box, with lights on and eyes open.
- Looking at the lights is not recommended; rather, people are free to engage in such activities as reading and writing, or eating meals.

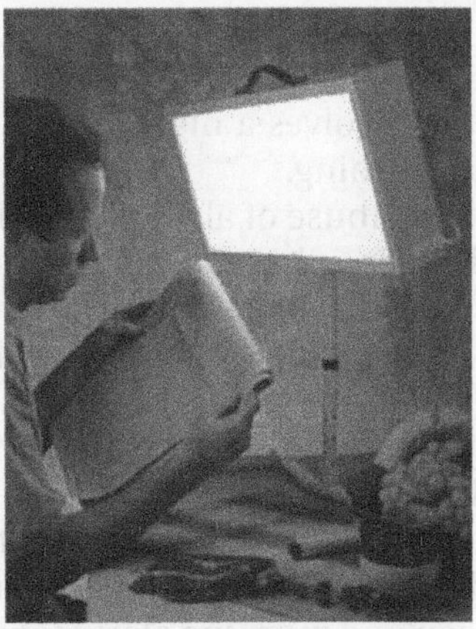

Figure 28.1: Exposure to light therapy

- What is important is to orient the head and body toward the lights, concentrating on activities on the surfaces illuminated by the lights, and not on the lights themselves.
- Treatment sessions can last from 15 minutes to three hours, once or twice a day, depending on individual needs and equipment used.

BENEFITS OF LIGHT THERAPY

- Increasingly, light therapy is being used to reset our body clocks—sometimes along with melatonin and sometimes on its own—no matter how or why they have been put off track.
- Scientists are discovering that light therapy may have potential for treatment of several other disorders in addition to that of SAD.

Early Morning Insomnia

- Those suffering from this illness, find that they cannot sleep in the early morning.
- In a 1993 study conducted at South Australia, 9 persons who have suffered from early morning insomnia underwent bright-light stimulation in the evening.
- They were given phototherapy that involved exposure to 2,500 lux light from 10 pm to midnight. The result— They fell asleep at their normal times; but, stayed asleep an average of one and a half hours longer than usual.

Productivity Enhancement

A study in Wetaskiwin, Alberta, Canada, clearly showed that students in classrooms with full-spectrum light had less absenteeism and had a higher academic-achievement than students in classes conducted under ordinary fluorescent lighting.

Night-owl Insomnia

- One type of insomnia involves a nightly inability to fall asleep until the wee hours of the morning.
- This often results in the abuse of alcohol and sleeping pills.
- It's called delayed sleep phase syndrome (DSPS), or night-owl insomnia, and it usually develops during the teen years.
- Researchers blame it on having a maladjusted biological rhythm that doesn't say 'good-night' until several hours past a normal bedtime.
- In one study of people suffering from delayed sleep-phase syndrome, light therapy involving two hours of bright-light exposure in the morning and then restriction from bright-light in the evening hours, successfully altered the troubled sleepers' circadian rhythms.
- In addition, both sleep and morning alertness improved significantly during the treatment.

Jet Lag

- Some people have been able to avoid, or at least minimize the effect of, jet lag with light therapy.
- Experts recommend that if you are planning a trip eastward-to Europe, for example—you may want to try to get up a few hours earlier than normal, on the day you intend to fly.
- Take a walk and soak up the sun, or stay inside with all the lights on. Stay awake and surround yourself with light.
- Then, once you arrive at your destination, try to stay outside in the sun for an hour or two. By doing so, you may be able to move your clock forward to more closely match the rhythm of life in the new time zone.

Late-shift Drowsiness

- According to the National Commission of Sleep Disorders Research, people who work nights are two to five times more likely to fall asleep on the job and have accidents.
- Late-night sleepiness may impair the judgment of police, firefighters and ambulance drivers. In addition, a disturbing number of airline disasters have occurred in the wee hours.
- In an analysis of ten studies involving nightshift workers, researchers found that the circadian rhythms of the subjects could be successfully shifted after bright-light exposure at night and complete darkness during the day for four days.
- These shifts resulted in significant improvement in both alertness and cognitive performance during work hours. In addition, the workers were able to sleep an average of two hours longer during the day.

Bulimia

- This binge/purge eating disorder typically develops in women during their teenage or early adult years.
- If bulimia remains untreated, it can cause serious physical and emotional problems.
- Some researchers have noted that bulimic episodes seem to occur most frequently in winter, leading to speculation that the illness might have a seasonal component.
- People who underwent high intensity light therapy had shown a remarkable improvement in this condition.

Lupus

- Lupus is an autoimmune disease meaning that the immune system mistakes the body's own tissues for germs and attacks them.

- It strikes many more women than men and can cause a confusing array of symptoms, including fatigue, rashes, joint pains and kidney damage.
- People with lupus are usually warned to avoid sunlight because it can aggravate their symptoms. But scientists have discovered that one type of ultraviolet sunlight, UVA-1, helps relieve lupus symptoms.

Nonseasonal Depression

- Some 10–15 million Americans are seriously depressed, and the suicide claims 30,000 lives a year.
- The success of light therapy in treating SAD has led to studies of its effectiveness for nonseasonal depression with promising preliminary results.

Prolonged Menstrual Cycles

- The typical menstrual cycle lasts about a month, but some women's extend upto twice as long.
- In a study, a number of women who suffered from prolonged menstrual cycles were asked to sleep with a 100 Watt light on for five nights near the middle of their extended cycles.
- The results were amazing. Their cycles became shorter.
- Scientists speculate that the light might be affecting the regulation of female sex hormones. If so, phototherapy might one day be used to treat some cases of infertility.

Chapter 29 Color Therapy

INTRODUCTION

Color therapy, also known as chromotherapy, is often facilitated in the healing rooms of alternative health practitioners. Color therapy is classified as a vibrational healing modality. *Vibrational medicine* incorporates the use of chi energies within living organisms such as plants, gemstones and crystals, water, sunlight, and sound.

Color is simply a form of visible light, of electromagnetic energy. All the primary colors reflected in the *rainbow* carry their own unique healing properties. The sun alone is a wonderful healer! Just imagine what life would be like without sunshine. It has been proven that lack of sunlight contributes to depression for some people.

Color therapy (also known as *chromotherapy*) is an exciting new form of healing brought forward from the Atlantean teachings, and is complementary to such modalities as kinesiology, acupuncture and other natural healing modalities.

BACKGROUND

- Chromotherapy is a therapeutic science which has been used by many races for thousands of years.
- The ancient Egyptians used specially built solarium rooms with different colored glasses.
- The sun would shine through the colored glass onto the patient to achieve specific therapeutic benefits. Others used different colored silk clothes to filter varying shades of light onto their bodies.
- There is also evidence of others using colored waters and colored gels to achieve the same results.
- These days, many natural therapists are using chromotherapy on their patients in interesting ways.
- They report success in recovery of stroke victims, and in others who have chronic depression.

HEALING POWER OF COLOR THERAPY

- Find treatment for physical and mental problems like:
  - Seasonal affective disorder (SAD)

- High blood pressure
- Headache
- Depression
- Colds and flu
- Stress and fatigue
- Memory and brain disorder
- In proper circulation, heart diseases and respiratory conditions
- Body aches and stiffness
- Skin conditions, and more.

- Achieve personal and spiritual growth with these sessions: Creating wealth and career opportunities, attracting your soul mate, improving your love life and personal relationships. Or, if you wish, you can create your own session—A sequence of colors you choose to address your specific symptoms.
- Easy to use no need to stare directly at the computer screen—Just playing the session in the same room will provide the same benefits (remember, color and light are energy).
- Receive interlight color therapy treatment benefits while relaxing, watching TV, reading, or have one running in a background computer window while you work.
- Enhance and strengthen mental power and creativity during social or business gatherings, classes and meetings with a special color therapy session.
- Use any of our sessions as often as you like—Your instant online membership give you access to the sessions you need when you need them.
- Completely safe noninvasive and nontoxic can be safely used as an alternative therapy or as a complementary therapy to conventional medicine to enhance its effectiveness.
- Convenient to use at work, at home, or anywhere in the world there's Internet access. You'll never need to visit a spa or wellness center to receive the benefits of color light therapy.

TOOLS USED IN COLOR THERAPY

- Gemstones
- Candles/lamps
- Crystal wands
- Crystal and glass prisms
- Colored fabrics
- Color bath treatments
- Colored eye lenses
- Lasers.

BENEFITS OF COLOR THERAPY

- Color therapy has innumerable benefits which are often misunderstood.

- Color therapy is useful in raising the energy levels of a person considerably.
- Each color has a particular property and tendency; they can be used according to the needs and mood of a person.

THE MEANING AND POWER OF COLOR

RED is hot. It can stimulate and excite. It connects to our physical self.

Red is associated with:	*Benefits may be:*	*Too much red may result in:*
• Courage • Strength • Vitality • Vigor • Ambition • Alertness • Sexuality • Pioneering spirit • Willpower • Aggressiveness	• Overcoming negative thoughts • A sense of power • Self-confidence • Settledness • A feeling of security and safety • Appetite stimulant • Possible Tourette syndrome cure	• Impatience • Increase aggressiveness • Hostility • Irritation • Anger

ORANGE is warm and joyful. It connects to our emotional self.

Orange is associated with:	*Benefits may be:*	*Too much orange may result in:*
• Sociability • Social confidence • Success • Happiness • Resourcefulness	• Optimism • Cheering • Antidepressant • Inspiring • Expanded interest and activities • Enjoyable relationships • Help remove inhibitions	• Irritability • Slight frustration • Increased appetite

YELLOW is warm to hot. It connects to our mental self.

Yellow is associated with:	*Benefits may be:*	*Too much yellow may result in:*
• Mental clarity • Cheerfulness • Optimism • Self-esteem	• Memory • Concentration • Stimulating curiosity and interest • Easing of depression	• Superficiality • Hyperactivity

Contd...

Contd...

Yellow is associated with:	*Benefits may be:*	*Too much yellow may result in:*
• Wisdom • Inspiration	• Empowerment • Confidence • Courage • Helps with anxiety • Energy • Aids discriminant and decision-making	

GREEN is the master color. It is refreshing and cool. It connects us to unconditional love.

Green is associated with:	*Benefits may be:*	*Too much green may result in:*
• Peace • Renewal • Love • Hope • Balance • Harmony • Self-control • Growth • Life	• Stress reduction • Rest • Calmness • Sense of balance and normalcy • Relaxation	• Laziness

AQUA (turquoise) is cooling. It connects us to our expression.

Aqua is associated with:	*Benefits may be:*	*Too much aqua may result in:*
• Purity • Soothing feeling • Calmness • Confidence • Oratory • Openness	• Relaxation • Loving expressiveness • Freedom of expression • Help with sleep • Sensitivity	• None known

BLUE is cold and acidic. It connects us to holistic thoughts.

Blue is associated with:	*Benefits may be:*	*Too much blue may result in:*
• Communication • Creativity	• Mental relaxation • Calmness • Peace	• Insecurity • Pessimism

Contd...

Contd...

Blue is associated with:	*Benefits may be:*	*Too much blue may result in:*
• Personal expression • Vitality • Decisiveness • Knowledge • Health	• Help with insomnia • Confidence in speaking • Clear communication • Help with hyperactivity in children	• Feel tired • Depressed • Cold-natured

INDIGO is cool and calming to the nervous system. It connects us to our unconscious self.

Indigo is associated with:	*Benefits may be:*	*Too much indigo may result in:*
• Serenity • Stillness • Imagination • Understanding	• Imagination • Greater intuition and awareness • Accurate perception • Strong, deep sleep	• Depression • Sense of separateness from others

VIOLET is cool. It connects us to our spiritual self.

Violet is associated with:	*Benefits may be:*	*Too much violet may result in:*
• Inspiration • Creativity • Beauty	• Generosity • Selflessness • Enhanced artistic ability • Strong, deep sleep • Calm nerves • Reduced excitement • Reduced irritation • Suppress appetite	• Depression • Insecurity • Stagnate or suppress emotions (especially anger)

MAGENTA is balancing. It connects us to devotional love.

Magenta is associated with:	*Benefits may be:*	*Too much magenta may result in:*
• Soothing • Relaxing • Gentle	• Balance of emotions for both the over and under emotional • Peace	• Can be too relaxing (not good for the introverted or chronically depressed)

Baker-Miller PINK is relaxing. Read more about Baker-Miller PINK

Baker-Miller PINK is associated with:	*Baker-Miller PINK may be:*	*Too much Baker-Miller PINK may result in:*
• Relaxation • Stress relief • Calming aggression	• An appetite suppressant	• There are no known results from an overdose of Baker-Miller PINK • Read more about *Baker-Miller PINK*

WHITE:

Used for regeneration: Also, provides energy and balances the chronobiological rhythm, by stimulating the production of serotonin, a substance which regulates both sleep and the nervous system.

Rebalances the psychophysical and hormonal systems in people who suffer from seasonal depression.

GOLD:

Esoteric/magical: Absolute authority, (self) confidence, creativity, perfection, solar energies, male energy, financial riches, investments, luxury, winning, worldly power, magical power, overcoming bad habits/ addictions.

SILVER:

Esoteric/magical: Female energy, cycles, rebirth, reincarnation, healing of hormonal imbalances, emotional stability, remove or neutralize negativity, intuition, dreams, psychic abilities and psychic workings.

COPPER/BRONZE:

Esoteric/magical: Love and passion, for positive relationships in love, friendship and business, career promotions, negotiations.

RESEARCH REVIEW

Depression: A study commissioned by the American Psychiatric Association and led by a psychiatrist at the University of North Carolina at Chapel Hill School of Medicine has found that:

Light therapy effectively treats mood disorders, including seasonal affective disorder (SAD) and other depressive disorders. A report of the study, which appeared in the American Journal of Psychiatry, also finds that the effects of light therapy, also known as phototherapy, are comparable to those found in many clinical studies of antidepressant drug therapy for these disorders.

Chapter 30 Aromatherapy

INTRODUCTION

Aromatherapy is the ancient science of healing, relaxing and energizing by the use of plants and their parts. The roots, barks, flowers, fruits, seeds and nuts play a crucial part in this science. It is one of the more popular branches of alternative medicines.

- The word aromatherapy is derived from two words 'aroma' which means smell and 'therapy' which stands for healing.
- *Essential oils* form the basis of aromatherapy.
- These essentials oils are the extracts of plants and their parts and form their life force.
- These oils are extracted by the means of steam distillation, cold expression, or fixed oil or alcohol extraction.
- They are highly concentrated and should not be used directly.
- These oils can be blended together and this blend is called synergy.
- The synergy is more potent than the individual oils combined.
- To reduce the potency of these oils, you can dilute them by mixing them with carrier oils.
- These oils affect your mood. They enter through our olfactory system and affect the nervous system, thus improving mood and relaxing or energizing us.

This helps is alleviating stress and speeding up healing. These essential oils also have cosmetic properties and can be used in skin care and hair care products. Many of these oils have known antiviral, antifungal and antiseptic properties. They are also used in household products for cleaning and antiseptic uses.

These oils can be inhaled, massaged onto your body, added to the bath or shower or sprayed in the room. The essential oils used in aromatherapy are the life force of the plants from which they have been extracted. These oils can be massaged on your body, inhaled, added to your bath or sprayed in the air. When you take *Aromatherapy massage* with the essential oils, these oils are absorbed into the bloodstream via the skin.

HOW DOES AROMATHERAPY WORK?

- Researchers are not entirely clear how aromatherapy may work. Some experts believe our sense of smell may play a role.

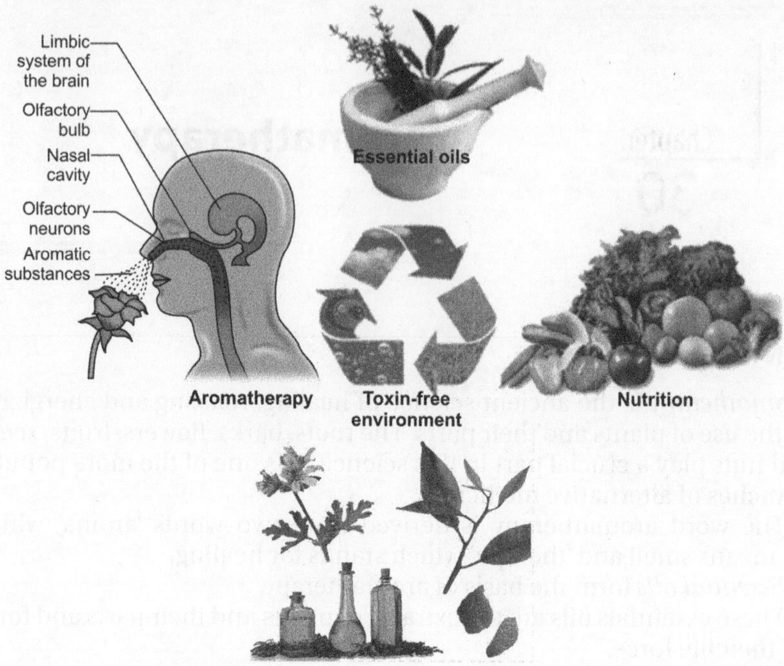

Figure 30.1: Contents of aromatherapy

- The 'smell' receptors in your nose communicate with parts of your brain (the amygdala and hippocampus) that serve as storehouses for emotions and memories.
- When you breathe in essential oil molecules, some researchers believe that they stimulate these parts of your brain and influence physical, emotional, and mental health. For example, lavender is believed to stimulate the activity of brain cells in the amygdala similar to the way some sedative medications work.
- Other researchers think that some molecules from essential oils may interact in the blood with hormones or enzymes.
- Aromatherapy massage is a popular way of using essential oils because it works in several ways at the same time. Your skin absorbs essential oils and you also breathe them in. Plus, you experience the physical therapy of the massage itself.

WHAT HAPPENS DURING AN AROMATHERAPY SESSION? (FIG. 30.1)

- Professional aromatherapists, nurses, physical therapists, pharmacists, and massage therapists can provide topical or inhaled aromatherapy treatment.
- Only specially trained professionals can provide treatment that involves taking essential oils by mouth.

- At an aromatherapy session, the practitioner will ask about your medical history and symptoms, as well as any scents you may like.
- You may be directed to breathe in essential oils directly from a piece of cloth or indirectly through steam inhalations, vaporizers, or sprays.
- The practitioner may also apply diluted essential oils to your skin during a massage. In most cases, the practitioner will tell you how to use aromatherapy at home, by mixing essential oils into your bath.

WHAT IS AROMATHERAPY GOOD FOR?

- Aromatherapy is used in a wide range of settings—from health spas to hospitals — to treat a variety of conditions. In general, it seems to
  - relieve pain
  - improve mood and
  - promote a sense of relaxation.
- Several clinical studies suggest that when essential oils (particularly rose, lavender, and frankincense) were used by qualified midwives, pregnant women felt less anxiety and fear, had a stronger sense of well-being, and had less need for pain medications during delivery.
- Many women also report that peppermint oil relieves nausea and vomiting during labor.
- Massage therapy with essential oils (combined with medications or therapy) may benefit people with depression. The scents are thought by some to stimulate positive emotions in the area of the brain responsible for memories and emotions, but the benefits seem to be related to relaxation caused by the scents and the massage.
- A person's belief that the treatment will help also influences whether it works.
- In test tubes, chemical compounds from some essential oils have shown antibacterial and antifungal properties.
- Some evidence also suggests that citrus oils may strengthen the immune system and that peppermint oil may help with digestion.
- Fennel, aniseed, sage, and clary-sage have estrogen-like compounds, which may help relieve symptoms of premenstrual syndrome and menopause. However, human studies are lacking.

OTHER CONDITIONS FOR WHICH AROMATHERAPY MAY BE HELPFUL INCLUDES

- Alopecia areata (hair loss)
- Agitation, possibly including agitation related to dementia
- Anxiety
- Constipation (with abdominal massage using aromatherapy)
- Insomnia
- Pain: Studies have found that people with rheumatoid arthritis, cancer (using topical chamomile), and headaches (using topical peppermint) require fewer pain medications when they use aromatherapy

- Itching, a common side effect for those receiving dialysis
- Psoriasis
- Stress
- Muscular aches and pains
- Headaches
- Digestive problems
- Menstrual or menopausal problems.

AVOID AROMATHERAPY

- Pregnant women, people with severe asthma, and people with a history of allergies should avoid all essential oils.
- Pregnant women and people with a history of seizures should avoid hyssop oil.
- People with high blood pressure should avoid stimulating essential oils such as rosemary and spike lavender.
- People with estrogen-dependent tumors (such as breast or ovarian cancer) should not use oils with estrogen-like compounds such as fennel, aniseed, sage, and clary-sage.
- People receiving chemotherapy should talk to their doctor before trying aromatherapy.

CONTRAINDICATION

Before using aromatherapy, you need to bear in mind that in their concentrated form the oils might be poisonous. You should handle them carefully and always dilute them according to the product instructions. Aromatherapy may not be appropriate for everyone. Take extra care if you have conditions including:

- Allergies
- Hay fever
- Asthma
- Eczema
- Sensitive skin.

Aromatherapy oils can have side effects. Side effects are the unwanted, but mostly mild and temporary effects of a treatment. Side effects of aromatherapy may include:

- Feeling sick
- Headaches
- Allergic reactions.

Some oils, including citrus ones such as orange, grapefruit and bergamot, react with ultraviolet light and can cause your skin to burn more easily in sunlight.

Don't use essential oils neat on your skin. Exceptions are lavender oil and tea-tree oil but only in small amounts and not for long periods. Applying lavender and tea-tree oils to the skin over a long period of time has been linked to breast enlargement in boys who haven't yet reached puberty. This is thought to be because the oils may act in a similar way to the female sex hormone, estrogen.

Don't use essential oils on broken skin. It is important not to swallow oils or apply them directly inside your body (e.g. inside your nostril or ear).

RESEARCH REVIEW

The Effects of Aromatherapy on Stress and Stress Responses in Adolescents

Purpose

This study was done to examine the effects of aromatherapy on stress and stress responses in adolescents.

Methods

A two-group crossover design was used for this study. The experimental treatment was aroma essential oil (using Bergamot essential oil) inhalation and the placebo treatment was carrier oil inhalation using a necklace. The sample included 36 female high school students. Fisher's exact test, t-test, and paired t-test using SPSS/WIN program were used to analyze the data.

Results

Stress levels were significantly lower when the students received the aroma treatment compared to when they received the placebo treatment. The stress responses except salivary IgA levels were significantly lower when the students received the aroma treatment.

Conclusion

Aroma inhalation could be a very effective stress management method for high school students. Therefore, it is recommended that this program be used in clinical practice as an effective nursing intervention for high school students.

BIBLIOGRAPHY

1. J Korean Acad Nurs. 2009 Jun;39(3):357-65. Seo JY. Department of Nursing, Youngnam Foreign Language College, Gyeongsan, Korea. marseo@hanmail.net.

Chapter 31

Spiritual Therapy

ABSTRACT

A state of wholeness or health is dependent not only on one's relationship to the physical and interpersonal environment but also to the spiritual aspects of self. The role of the spirit is healing, is witnessed in all cultures. Health care sciences have begins to demonstrate that spirituality, faith and religious commitment may play a role in promoting health and reducing illness. It is a core of many modalities.

HISTORICAL REVIEW

Throughout history, people have dealt with pain, illness and healing in spiritual ways. Ancient Babylonians and Egyptians performed elaborate healing rituals in temples. The ancient Greeks used dream including methods to treat various disorders.

DEFINITION

According to Milne (1984)—'Spirituality from a pastoral perspectives referring to a vital expression of a person total being the wholeness of the spirit'.

MODALITIES OF SPIRITUAL THERAPY

The term spirituality is derive from the latin word 'Spirace' means 'to breathe life', spirituality develops hopes and love.

1. *Faith Healing*: Faith healing is the practitioner's belief that one has to purify one's self and reach a state of unity with GOD or a high power.
2. *Healing Prayer*: Prayer is most often defined simply as a form of communication and fellowship with the creator. It is also defined as an 'active process of appealing to a higher spiritual power, specifically for health reasons'.

NURSES ROLE IN SPIRITUAL THERAPY

1. Nurses that the only patient with spiritual issues are those who articulate using such words as 'God', church and haven while religious life experiences as a significant part of one's personality.

2. Some spiritual issues are raised in anger and disbeliefs, e.g. why did God pick me, 'I don't deserve this end, I've live a good life'.
   The nurse support the patient and not to defend God and quietly acknowledge, therefore, Yes I don't understood either'.
3. Spiritual support may also take the form of sitting with the patient during a religious, ritual joining a prayer, reading or providing inspiration literature.
4. Nurses can only adequately provide the spiritual care if they have examined their own beliefs and discovered how the truths and religious principles have guided their own lives.

PRAYER THERAPY

Prayer is a petition, a request for peace, a demand for wholeness, a desire and need for problem solution, a way to give thanks, and to praise

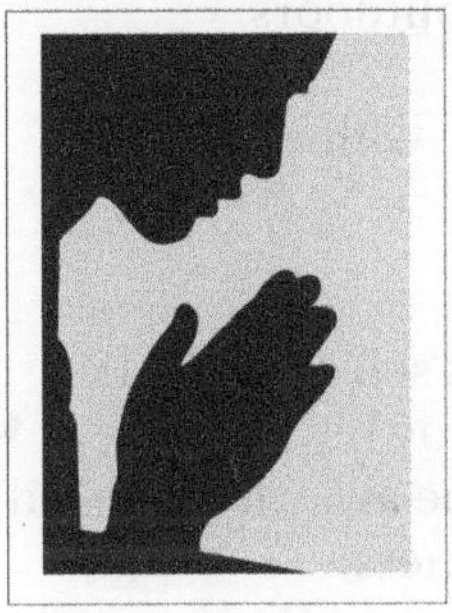

Figure 31.1: Prayer therapy

God expressed by words quietly or loudly and uttered in a humble way, begging the God who created human, who is capable of doing or making things possible, which is impossible, who is answer to all questions and who is a way to all strange highways in life (Fig. 31.1).

Prayer: An Effective Alternative Medicine Therapy

Prayer does affect healing and the outcome of illness even when the patient does not know they are being prayed for. This has been shown in many research studies over the past few years.

But should prayer be considered an alternative medicine therapy? The answer is yes, if you research the subject and the research study results over the past years.

Meaning of prayer

Prayer comes from French word 'Preier' means to request.

Prayer therapy is the practice of using prayer therapeutically in a clinical, intensive treatment and learning session for the purpose of emotional and mental healing and wholeness.

Prayer therapy engages the person's soul (mind, will, and emotions) in a conscience process of transformation; rather than just praying for them to be healed.

Ways of prayer

- Position:
  - — Sitting
  - — Kneel down
  - — Standing.
- Customary
  - — Once, twice, thrice....
  - — Before or after some actions.
- Individual
  - — Alone, with family or friends, in a group.
- Venue
  - — Close or open room, outdoors.
- Approach
  - — With tears, with smile, with clap.

Preparation before prayer

1. Caring attitude towards self and others
2. Contacting God by calling his name
3. Concentrating fully to be away from world
4. Ask pardon and forgiveness
5. Feeling the holly presence of God.

Steps of prayer

- Welcoming the arrival of God
- Prayer
- Meditation
- Visualization and self-retrospection
- Daily awakening
- Thanks giving.

Prayer practice

- Gently shift your attention to the area around your heart.
- Adjust your breathing in order that you are inhaling and exhaling in the heart and out by means of the solar plexus.
- Stimulate an authentic emotion of thanks or care for someone or something in your daily life.
- Generate a genuine effort to maintain emotions of gratitude, care or love while radiating them to one-self as well as others.
- Whenever you find your mind (attention) roaming or getting involved in negative thoughts and emotions, carefully focus your

inhaling and exhaling back again in the heart and solar plexus and reunite with genuine recitation of the Jesus Prayer.

BIBLIOGRAPHY

1. Carven, Ruth F. Fundamental of Nursing, 5th ed. Philadelplhia, Lippincott Williams and Wilkins. 2007; 1392 –5.
2. Ladner, C SUE: Fundamental of Nursing, 3rd ed. New York, Thomson Delmar; 300–25.
3. Nurses of India. Aug: 2007; Vol VIII, 4–6.

UNIT-V
Complementary and Alternative Therapies in Psychiatry

INTRODUCTION

An alternative approach to mental health care is one that emphasizes the interrelationship between mind, body, and spirit. Although some alternative approaches have a long history, many remain controversial. The National Center for Complementary and Alternative Medicine at the National Institutes of Health was created in 1992 to help evaluate alternative methods of treatment and to integrate those that are effective into mainstream health care practice. It is crucial, however, to consult with your health care providers about the approaches you are using to achieve mental wellness.

We face many circumstances in our journey of life. We also have to contend with issue such as aging and sickness. The desired of all human is good health. Good health is a treasure but not type of health induced by constant consumption of various tonics and medicines. The mainstream of health care (western allopathic medicine) mainly focusing the curing of the body. But alternative approaches to the health care are the focusing on the whole person and its view in holistic approach. It recognizes holism as interrelationship of biopsychological, spiritual dimension of the person and emphasis provide total person care.

ALTERNATIVE APPROACHES TO HEALTH CARE

The term alternative and complementary healing modalities was first articulated at the national level in 1996. These therapies are not accepted by mainstream conventional medical practices.

DEFINITION OF ALTERNATIVE THERAPY

- Alternative therapy is defined through a social process as those practices that do not form part of the dominant system for managing health and disease.
- An unrelated group of nonorthodox practices often with explanatory system that do not follow conventional biomedical explanations.

COMPLEMENTARY THERAPIES

Therapeutic practices that are not currently considered and integral part of conventional allopathic medical practice.

So these practices and therapies that do not form part of the dominant system for managing health and disease are called alternative and complementary therapies.

BASIC CONCEPTS OF ALTERNATIVE HEALTH CARE

1. Mind and body are not separate. The whole system must be considered if the part of the individual are to be helped to function.
2. People are responsible for their own choices, person integrated and related to his or her surroundings.
3. People have the power to solve their own problems. There exists some life forces or energy that can be used in the healing process.
4. Well-being is multifaceted ritual, prescribed practice and skilled practitioners are integral part of holistic healing intervention.

CATEGORIES OF ALTERNATIVE THERAPIES

Alternative health care approaches are divided into two categories:

1. Traditional methods
2. Nontraditional methods.

TYPES OF ALTERNATIVE THERAPIES

There are different kinds of alternative therapies:

1. Diet management and nutrition
2. Animal assisted therapies
3. Ayurveda
4. Yoga/meditation
5. Massage therapy
6. Telemedicine
7. Herbal medicine
8. Siddha

9. Unani
10. Homeopathic
11. Acupuncture
12. Acupressure
13. Chiropractice medicine.

Diet Management and Nutrition

In last 40 years nutritional interventions for prevention and treatment of diseases have received increased interest from consumers and health care providers. The *Orthomolecular* diet embodies to principles of introducing the foods, that the body can use best in a manner that assist the digestion, absorption and utilization. It is very similar in many ways to what is referred to as the hunter gatherer diet, but embodies principles meant to help us survive in 20th century life. Here is the essence of the orthomolecular diet.

Adjusting both diet and nutrition may help some people with mental illnesses, manage their symptoms and promote recovery. For example, research suggests that eliminating milk and wheat products can reduce the severity of symptoms for some people who have schizophrenia and some children with autism. Similarly, some holistic/natural physicians use herbal treatments, B-complex vitamins, riboflavin, magnesium, and thiamine to treat anxiety, autism, depression, drug-induced psychoses, and hyperactivity.

Animal Assisted Therapies

In Britain in the 18th–19th centuries, pet were used in institutions to give a sense of meaning and purpose to people institutionalized because of developmental delays. Many health care professionals are finding that lonliness may be as serious as cancer and heart disease for older adults, playing with pet animal can help people feel less isolated. It is used for long-term and acute care setting help overcome physical limitations. Improve mood, decrease blood pressure and improve socialization skill and self-esteem.

Working with an animal (or animals) under the guidance of a health care professional may benefit some people with mental illness by facilitating positive changes, such as increased empathy and enhanced socialization skills. Animals can be used as part of group therapy programs to encourage communication and increase the ability to focus. Developing self-esteem and reducing loneliness and anxiety are just some potential benefits of individual-animal therapy (Delta Society, 2002).

Ayurveda

Ayurveda is an ancient Hindu system is to maintain which originated in India. Its main goal is to maintain the health of unhealthy people and cure the illness of seeks people. Ayurveda maintain that illness is the result of falling out of balance with nature. Diagnosis is based on three metabolic body types call doshas. An ayurvedic doctor determines the dosha type as vata, pitta or kapha.

Treatment usually involves prescribing a diet, herbal remedies, breath work, physical exercises, yoga meditation, massage and a rejundenation or detoxification program.

Ayurveda is rapidly becoming more popular in America. The books and Vedas of Deepak Chopra are an example of this increasingly popular system of therapy.

Ayurvedic medicine is described as 'knowledge of how to live.' It incorporates an Individualized regimen—such as diet, meditation, herbal preparations, or other techniques—to treat a variety of conditions, including depression, to facilitate lifestyle changes, and to teach people how to release stress and tension through yoga or transcendental meditation.

Yoga/Meditation

The tradition of Yoga was born in India several thousand years ago. Maharishi Patanjali rightly called as the 'Father of Yoga'. Practitioners of this ancient Indian system of health care use breathing exercises, posture, stretches, and meditation to balance the body's energy centers. Yoga is used in combination with other treatment for depression, anxiety, and stress-related disorders.

Yoga discipline that focuses on the body musculature, posture, breathing mechanisms and consciousness.

Yoga is a method by which one can develop once inherent powers in a balanced manner. It offers the means to reach complete self-realizations. The literal meaning of the Sanskrit word yoga is to Yoke. 'Yoga can be defined as a means for uniting the individual spirit with the universal spirit'.

Types of yoga

1. Jap Yoga: People need to concentrate once mind on the divine or mantras like 'OM'.
2. Karma Yoga: People use to perform all actions without having and desires for there fruit.

3. Gyan Yoga: People wants to discriminate between the self and the nonself and to acquire the knowledge of ones spiritual entity through the study of scripture, saints and practice of medicine.
4. Hatha Yoga: Person purifies and stabilizes the body and vital energy, i.e. cleansing acts, diet regulation, asanas, pranayama, thereby acquire purity and stability of mind.
5. Bhakti Yoga: Bhakti yoga is a system of intense devotion with emphases on complete divine will, i.e. free from egonism, unaffected by the qualities of the world.
6. Raja Yoga: Ashtanga yoga is for the all around development of human personality.

Yamas (observences)

Practice of Yamas helps one to increase the power of concentration, mental purity and steadiness.

1. Ahimsa (not to harm others)
2. Satya(to be fruitful)
3. Aalasya (not to steal)
4. Bramhacharya (to observe celibacy)
5. Aparigraha (not to possesss beyond actual needs).

Massage Therapy

The underlying principle of this approach is that rubbing, kneading, brushing, and tapping a person's muscles can help release tension and pent emotions. It has been used to treat trauma-related depression and stress. A highly unregulated industry, certification for massage therapy varies widely from state-to-state. Some states have strict guidelines, while others have none.

Telemedicine

Telemedicine generally refers to the use of communication and information technologies for the delivery of clinical care. It may be as simple as two health professionals discussing a case over the telephone, or as complex as using satellite technology and video-conferencing equipment to conduct a real-time consultation between medical specialists in two different countries. Plugging into video and computer technology is a relatively new innovation in health care. It allows both consumers and providers in remote or rural areas to gain access to mental health or specialty expertise. Telemedicine can enable consulting providers to speak to and observe patients directly. It also can be used in education and training programs for generalist clinicians.

Herbal Medicine

Nature cure is a way of life of which we find a number of references in the Vedas and other ancient texts. The morbid matter theory, concept of vital force and other concepts upon which nature cure is based are already available in old texts which indicate that these methods were widely practiced in ancient India. Nature cure believes that all the diseases arise due to accumulation of morbid matter in the body and if scope is given for its removal, it provides cure or relief. It also believes that the human body possesses inherent self-constructing and self-healing powers. The fundamental difference in nature cure with other systems is that its theory and practice are based on holistic view point whereas the later's approach is specific. Nature cure does not believe in the specific cause of disease and its specific treatment but takes into account the totality of factors responsible for diseases such as one's unnatural habits in living, thinking, working, sleeping, relaxation, sexual indulgence, etc. and also considers the environmental factors involved which on the whole disturbs the normal functioning of the body and lead it to a morbid, weak and toxic state. For treatment it primarily stresses on correcting all the factors involved and allowing the body to recover itself. A nature cure physician helps in nature's effort to overcome disease by applying correct natural modalities and controlling the natural forces to work within safe limits. The five main modalities of treatment are air, water, heat, mud and space.

Siddha

Siddha system is one of the oldest systems of medicine in India. The term siddha means achievements and siddhas were saintly persons who achieved results in medicine. Eighteen siddhas were said to have contributed towards the development of this medical system. Siddha literature is in Tamil and it is practiced largely in Tamil-speaking part of India and abroad. The siddha system is largely therapeutic in nature. According to this system the human body is the replica of the Universe and so are the food and drugs irrespective of their origin.

The siddha system of medicine was its origin to the Dravidian culture. Which is the prevedic period, siddha system of medicine is mainly therapeutic, mercury, sulfur, iron, copper, gold bitumen, white, red and yellow arsenic and other material as well as vegetable poison are extensively used in siddha system.

This system believes that all objects in the Universe including human body are composed of five basic elements namely, earth, water, fire, air and sky. The food, which the human body takes and the drugs it uses are all, made of these five elements. The proportion of the elements present in the drugs vary and their preponderance or otherwise is responsible for certain actions and therapeutic results.

This system also deals with the concept of salvation in life. The exponents of this system consider achievement of this state is possible by medicines and meditation.

Uses of siddha

The system of siddha medicine is prevalent in southern states in India, Shri Lanka, Malaysia, Singapore where Dravidian civilization was dominant.

In north India the Siddha kalpa system is known as 'Tantrik Science'. In siddha system of medicine the first medical plant is 'Neem' tree which is used for smallpox and other infectious diseases and mental disorders.

Unani

Unani system of medicines originated in Greece and is based on the teachings of Hippocrates and Gallen and it developed into an elaborate Medical System by Arabs, like Rhazes, Avicenna, Al-Zahravi, Ibne-Nafis and others.

Unani Tibb or Graeco—Arab medicine may be traced to that system of Greek medicine developed during the Arab civilization. Muslims still call it unani medicine but European historians call it Arab medicine. It is practiced in the Indo-Pakistan subcontinent.

The basic framework consists of four humor theory of Hippocrates, i.e. blood, phlegm, yellow bile and black bile. Temperament occupies a very important place in unani Tibb and forms a basis of pathology, diagnosis and treatment. Disease is an expression of the imbalance of the humors or the disturbance to their harmony.

Unani medicines got enriched by imbibing what was best in the contemporary systems of traditional medicines in Egypt, Syria, Iraq, Persia, India, China and other Middle East countries. In India, Unani system of medicine was introduced by Arabs and soon it took firm roots. The Delhi Sultans (rulers) provided patronage to the scholars of Unani system and even enrolled some as state employees.

Unani system has shown remarkable results in curing the diseases like arthritis, leukoderma, jaundice, liver disorders, nervous system disorders, bronchial asthma, and several other acute and chronic diseases where other systems have not been able to give desired response. Now the system has crossed national boundaries and is popular among the masses globally.

Unani treatment is based on its natural and remarkable diagnosis methods and is affordable. It is mainly dependent on the temperament (Mizaj) of the patient, hereditary condition and effects, different complaints, signs and symptoms of the body, external observation, examination of the PULSE (Nubz), urine and stool, etc. Unique and special treatment methods like dietotherapy (Ilaj-bil-Ghiza), climatic therapy (Ilaj-bil-Hawa), regimental therapy (Ilaj-bit-Tadbir), make it a different and remarkable and popular system.

Concept of unani system

Unani Tibb seeks the restoration of the body as a whole to its original state. Unani system of treatment places great reliance on defense mechanism of the body. In times of epidemics, every precaution in maintaining a balance in diet and general health habits is recommended. In the classical literature of Tibb. There are certain prescription and prophylactic measures against the spread of infections, contagious diseases. Practitioners hold a respectable place in the society. The pharmacopeia consist of natural drugs mainly herbals but also includes animal, mineral and marine drugs. The drugs are used singly or in the form of infusion, powder, confections syrup and aqua's.

Homeopathy

Homeopathy, or homeopathic medicine, is a holistic system of treatment that originated in the late eighteenth century. The name homeopathy is derived from two Greek words that mean 'like disease.' The system is based on the idea that substances that produce symptoms of sickness in healthy people will have a curative effect when given in very dilute quantities to sick people who exhibit those same symptoms. Homeopathic remedies are believed to stimulate the body's own healing processes. Homeopaths use the term 'allopath,' or 'different than disease,' to describe the use of drugs used in conventional medicine to oppose or counteract the symptom being treated.

Homeopathy was founded by German physician Samuel Hahnemann (1755–1843), who was much disturbed by the medical system of his time, believing that its cures were crude and some of its strong drugs and treatments did more harm than good to patients. Hahnemann performed experiments on himself using Peruvian bark, which contains quinine, a *malaria* remedy. He concluded that in a healthy person, quinine creates the same symptoms as malaria, including fevers and chills, which is the reason why it is effective as a remedy. He then began to analyze the remedies available in nature by what he called proving. Proving of homeopathic remedies are still compiled by dosing healthy adults with various substances and documenting the results, in terms of the dose needed to produce the symptoms and the length of the dose's effectiveness. The proving are collected in large homeopathic references called Materia Medica or materials of medicine.

Acupuncture

The Chinese practice of inserting needles into specific points (acupoints) along the 'meridians' of the body and manipulated to relieve the discomfort associated with painful disorders, to induce surgical anesthesia, and for preventive and therapeutic purposes. It is proposed that acupuncture produces its effects by the conduction of electromagnetic signals at a greater-than-normal rate, thus aiding the activity of pain-killing biochemicals, such as endorphins and immune system cells, at specific sites in the body. Studies have also shown that acupuncture may alter brain chemistry by changing the release of neurotransmitters and neurohormones and affecting sensory perception and involuntary body functions. In recent years, the techniques have been adapted for use in veterinary medicine.

The traditional Chinese medicines claim to be to tell much about the patients checking pulses, looking at the color of the tongue checking facial color, assessing voice and smell and asking a variety of questions. To treat patients acupuncturists insert one or more needles along the medicines where flows, many acupuncturists also prescribes herbs.

Electroacupuncture

Electroacupuncture is a hand-held battery operated electronic device for self-relief through direct stimulation of pain, aches, tensions and stress-related insomnia. This stimulation can also serve to realize and enhance body energy level. Electroacupuncture is based on modern space technology coupled with the 4000 years old Chinese health care science of acupuncture.

Electroacupuncture is completely noninvasive, state of art method that replaces the classic acupuncture needle with electronic pulse stimulation. Stimulation is carried with 36 gold-plated conductive pulse pins. In addition, the biofeedback capability solves problem of correct application by locating the exact point to be stimulated. The user simply applies the device identifies the exact spot by detecting the low resistance points that are a critical mechanism in organic and natural pain relief. The pulse pin then send an electronic signal to the identified spot on the body.

Uses of electroacupuncture

Electroacupuncture is an effective in providing relief for a wide variety of pain conditions, including migraine and tension headaches, aching muscles and muscle strain, stress and stress-related insomnia back shoulder, elbow and knee pain, mood disorders.

Acupressure

Acupressure is a form of touchtherapy that utilizes the principles of acupuncture and Chinese medicine. In acupressure, the same points on the body are used as in acupuncture, but are stimulated with finger pressure. Acupressure is practiced as a treatment by Chinese medicine practitioners and acupuncturists, as well as by massage therapists. In massage therapy, acupressurists will evaluate a patient's symptoms and overall health, but a massage therapist's diagnostic training isn't as extensive as a Chinese physician's. In a massage therapy treatment, a person usually lies down on a table or mat, with thin clothing on. The acupressurist will gently feel and palpate the abdomen and other parts of the body to determine energy imbalances. Then, the therapist will work with different meridians throughout the body, depending on which organs are imbalanced in the abdomen. The therapist will use different types of finger movements and pressure on different acupoints, depending on whether the chi needs to be increased or dispersed at different points. The therapist observes and guides the energy flow through the patient's body throughout the session. Sometimes, special herbs (Artemesia vulgaris or moxa) may be placed on a point to warm it, a process called moxibustion. A session of acupressure is generally a very pleasant experience, and some people experience great benefit immediately. For more chronic conditions, several sessions may be necessary to relieve and improve conditions.

Chiropractic Medicine

Daniel David Palmer founded chiropractic in 1895. Chiropractic holds that illness is a result of nerve dysfunction. The main treatment modality of chiropractic is manipulation of the vertebral column and extremities. The goal is to remove the interference with the nerve functions so the body can heal itself, chiropractic do not perform surgery or drugs.

Chiropractic is a health care approach that focuses on the relationship between the body's structures mainly the spine and its functioning. Although practitioners may use a variety of treatment approaches, they primarily perform adjustments to the spine or other parts of the body with the goal of correcting alignment problems and supporting the body's natural ability to heal itself.

Chiropractic is from Greek words meaning 'done by hand'. It is grounded in the principle that the body can heal itself when the skeletal system is correctly aligned and the nervous system is functioning properly. To achieve this, the practitioner uses his or her hands or an adjusting tool to perform specific manipulations of the vertebrae. When these bones of the spine are not correctly articulated, resulting in a condition known as subluxation, the theory is that nerve transmission is disrupted and causes pain and illness manifested in the back as well as other areas of the body.

Chiropractic is one of the most popular alternative therapies currently available. Some would say it now qualifies as mainstream treatment as opposed to complementary medicine. Chiropractic treatment is covered by many insurance plans. It has become well-accepted treatment for acute pain and problems of the spine, including lower back pain and whiplash. Applications beyond that scope are not supported by current evidence, although there are ongoing studies into the usefulness of chiropractic for such problems as ear infections, dysmenorrhea, infant colic, migraine headaches, and other conditions.

THERAPEUTIC TOUCH

Delores Krieger, RN, PhD, and Dora Kunz, a natural healer, developed Therapeutic Touch (TT) in the early 1970s. TT is an adaptation of several religious and secular healing traditions and is commonly used in nursing practice for many different conditions.

TT practitioners hold their hands a short distance from the patient without actually making physical contact. The purpose of this technique is to detect the patient's energy field, allowing the TT practitioner to correct any perceived imbalances. Nurse Healers Professional Associates, Inc. is the primary training organization for Therapeutic Touch and teaches a standardized technique. TT treatment consists of four steps: centering (calming the mind and focusing attention on the patient), assessing the patient's energy field for irregularities, intervention to facilitate symmetrical flow of energy through the field, and evaluation/closure to verify the effects and conclude the treatment. Treatment sessions usually last from five to thirty minutes. Currently there is a lack of formal certification or competency-based assessment for this therapy.

The concept of 'life energy' or 'life force' has sometimes been compared to spiritual rather than scientific principles. Some critics argue that because of its religious roots, TT should be treated as a religion rather than as a health care therapy. Skeptics have sought to eliminate Therapeutic touch as a nursing practice, due to questions surrounding the mechanism of action. However, suggestive results from several human studies, positive clinical experience, and case reports have led to increasing use of TT.

Several variations have emerged from the original treatment but aspects of centering and intent have remained the foundations of this technique. Janet Mentgen founded healing touch in the 1980s based on the principles of therapeutic touch. Healing touch adds patient empowerment, practitioner self-care, and focuses on the impact of the practitioner-patient relationship. Therapeutic touch claims origin in ancient *energy healing* methods. Practitioners, primarily nurses, are trained to feel or sense energy imbalances in the patient's body, and to use 'laying on' of hands to disperse blocks and channel healing forces to the patient's body. This therapy shares a similar ideology to the energy zones in *reiki,* and how they are infused with good energy for healing. The therapist uses a light touch or holds his/her hands above the body; the client is usually seated in a *massage chair.* The therapist uses meditation to identify the energy field around a patient's body, and then to center and strengthen the connection to the patient's energy field using their hands. The therapist does this by scanning the body from head to toe. Their hands are typically held in a horizontal position, side by side with their thumbs touching and their palms facing the patient in a butterfly-like shadow. Again, there is no direct touch between healer and patient. The practitioner will sense the blockages in the body in hot and cold sensations.

Therapeutic touch is considered safe because of its gentle, noninvasive approach. The therapist actually rarely makes contact with the body at all. Therapeutic touch has been applied in an assortment of medical situations, including the care of premature infants, the healing of extensive wounds and the healing of emergency room patients. It is known to induce a state of relaxation within mere minutes.

Because each therapeutic touch session is different—The practitioner will use techniques specific to the client's needs—It is hard to describe what occurs. However many advocates of the treatment claim the following benefits:

- A sensation of enveloping warmth from the therapist's touch
- A totally relaxed state
- The feeling of vibrations of energy coursing through the entire body
- Intense euphoria and feelings of peace
- A kaleidoscope of color and beautiful light
- An intense sense of clarity, inner peace and well-being.

REIKI THERAPY

Reiki therapy is a technique for stress reduction and relaxation which involves the channelling of universal life force energy through the Reiki Practitioner by means of placing hands onto the recipient, with the intention of correcting any imbalance of energy.

Because the practitioner merely acts as a channel for the energy, he or she also benefits from the reiki energy as it passes through them!

Reiki works on the physical, emotional, mental and spiritual levels which means that, unlike orthodox medicine, it treats the person as a whole, rather than just the symptoms of a condition. The human body has a natural propensity to heal itself and reiki simply accelerates this process.

- Reiki is therefore 'universal life force energy' (Fig. V.1).

It is also the same energy known to many ancient civilizations, by many names, including Chi (Chinese), Prana (Asian Indian), Ruach

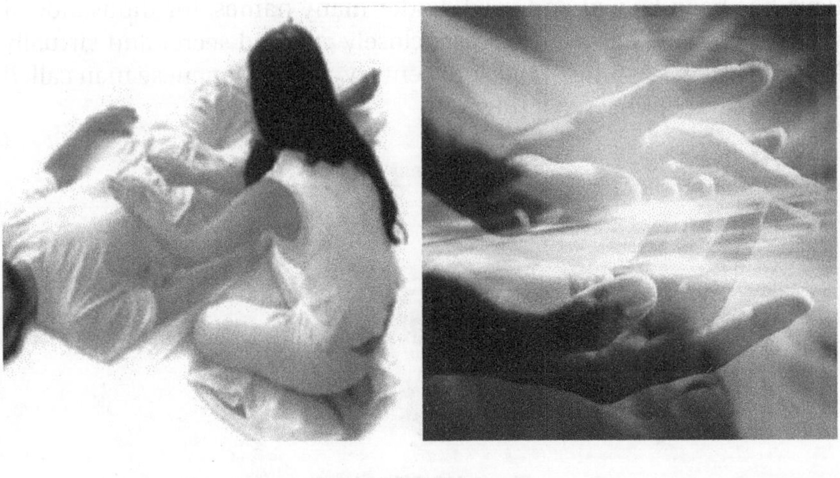

Figure V.1: Reiki therapy

(Hebrews), Mana (Polynesians) and Orenda (Iroquois Native Americans), to name but a few! reiki has been known and used, under many names, for thousands of years in the East but was kept as a closely guarded secret and virtually lost until the beginning of the 20th century, when a Japanese man called Mikao Usui rediscovered it.

The word 'Reiki' ('Rei-ki') is made up of two Japanese words:

'Rei'— Meaning 'universal, spiritual or free flowing'	REI 霊
and	
'Ki' — Meaning 'life force energy'	KI 気

There are many versions of the story of how reiki was rediscovered but they are not as important as the fact that it was found again! Most of the accounts state that Usui was searching for the healing methods used by great healers such as Jesus and Buddha. He eventually found the secret in the ancient Mahayana Sutras, the doctrine of life held sacred by Indian and Tibetan Buddhists.

This universal life force energy, by definition, is found everywhere in the Universe and is the same energy that modern science in general, and quantum physics in particular, recognizes as the subatomic energy which underlies all matter.

Although this energy is present everywhere, imbalances can and do occur. When they occur in the human body the results may include stress, inability to concentrate, depression and physical disease.

Reiki History

Reiki has been known and used, under many names, for thousands of years in the East but was kept as a closely guarded secret and virtually lost until the beginning of the 20th century, when a Japanese man called Mikao Usui rediscovered it (Fig. V.2).

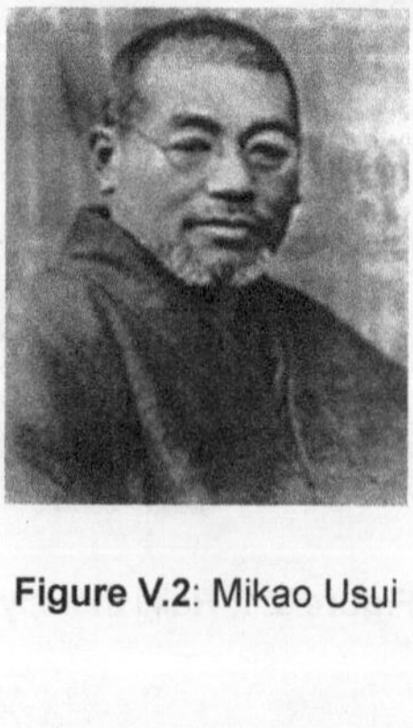

Figure V.2: Mikao Usui

Mikao Usui was born on August 15th, 1865, in the village of Yago. He was a, simple and humble person, physically healthy and well-proportioned. He never showed off and always had a smile on his face, he was also very courageous in the face of adversity. He was, at the same time, a very cautious person. He was a very talented student and travelled to several Western countries and China to study. He loved to read, and his knowledge of medicine, psychology, fortune telling and theology of religions around the world was vast. (It is also believed that he was well-versed in Ki Ko, the Japanese form of Chi Kung). It is unlikely that he was ever a Christian, as taught by Hawayo Takata, but he did study Tendai, Shingon, Mikkyo and Zen Buddhism.

At one point he did run into some bad luck (possibly a failed business venture) but he did not give up and trained himself arduously (Fig. V.3). In order to sort out his life he went to Mount Kurama, on a 21-day retreat to fast and meditate. It was at the end of this period that he felt the great

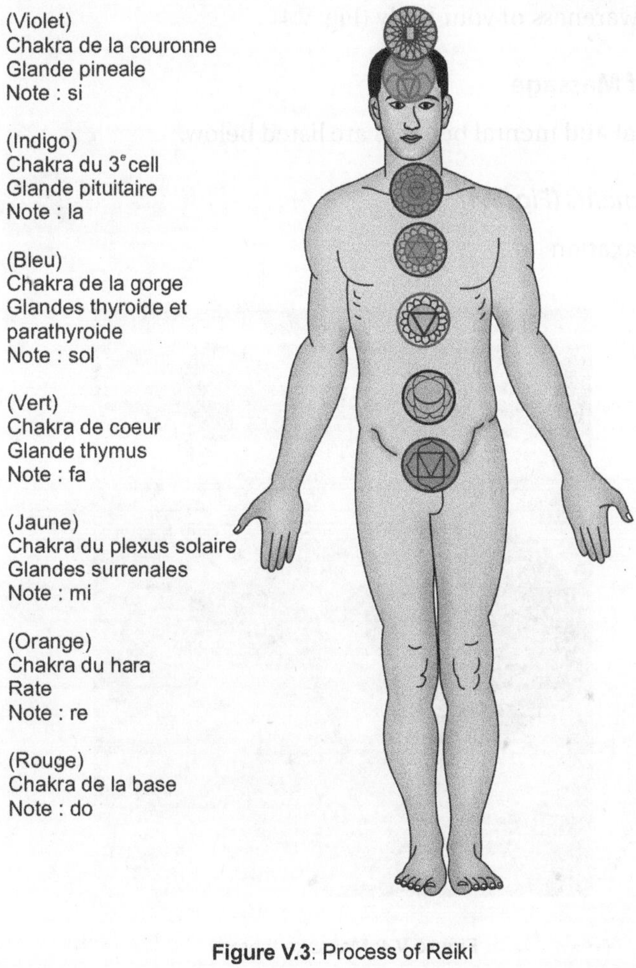

Figure V.3: Process of Reiki

Reiki energy over his head, which lead to the reiki healing system. He first used reiki on himself, then tried it on his family. Since it worked well for various ailments, he decided to share this knowledge with the public at large. He opened a clinic at Harajuku, Tokyo, in April 1922, where he not only gave treatment to many patients but also hosted workshops to spread his knowledge. Following the Kanto earthquake, in 1923, Usui took reiki to the devastated city and treated hundreds of the survivors. He became so popular that he had to open a new clinic at Nakano, in February 1925. He died from a stroke, in Fukuyama, on March 9th, 1926.

MASSAGE

Massage therapy can provide anything from soothing relaxation to deeper therapy for specific problems. It can relieve your stress and anxiety, increase the nourishing blood supply to your tissues, enhance your energy and alertness, and aid in your recovery from pulled muscles or sprained ligaments. Massage can also help with self-esteem and heighten awareness of your body (Fig. V.4).

Benefits of Massage

The physical and mental benefits are listed below.

Physical benefits (Fig. V.4)

- Aids relaxation

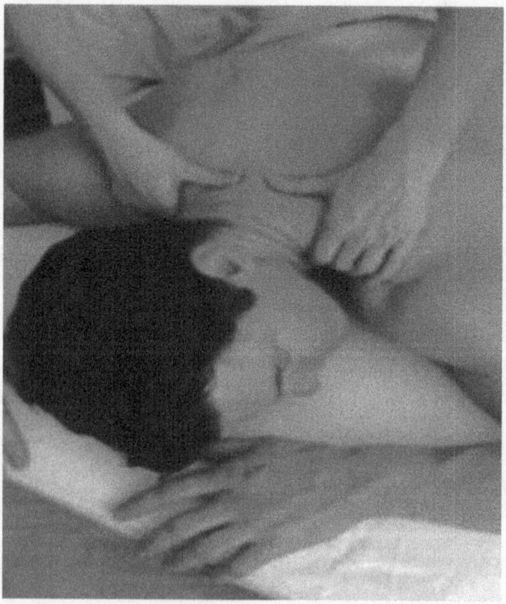

Figure V.4: Massage therapy

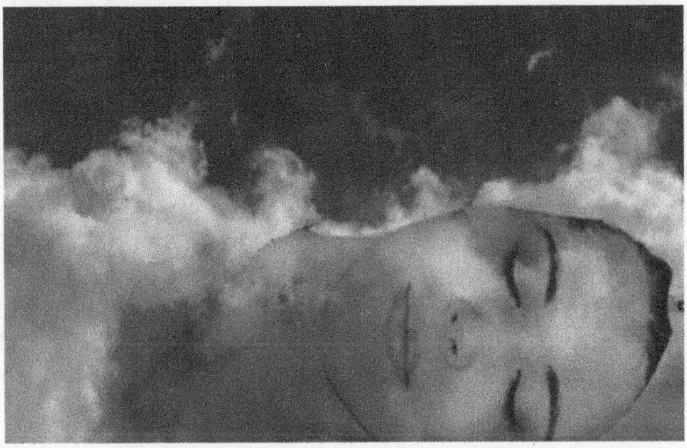

Figure V.5: Mental benefit of massage

- Helps relieve stress, muscle tension and stiffness
- Lightens discomfort during pregnancy
- Faster healing of strained muscles, sprained ligaments, swelling
- Reduce muscle spasms
- Provides greater flexibility and range of motion
- Enhances athletic performance
- Helps to deeper and easier breathing
- Improves blood circulation and movement of lymph fluids
- Reduce blood pressure
- Helps to relieve eye-strain and headaches caused by tension
- Enhances the health and nourishment of skin
- Improves posture
- Strengthens the immune system
- Rehabilitation after an operation or injury.

Mental benefits (Fig. V.5)

- Peace of mind and feeling of well-being
- Romotes a relaxed state of mental alertness
- Helps to relieve mental stress
- Improves ability to monitor stress signals and respond appropriately; calm thinking and creativity
- Emotional benefits.

MASSAGE-BASED THERAPIES TO IMPROVE WELL-BEING IN THE WORKPLACE

I work by combining my therapies to give clients a tailored massage to suit their particular condition. I have adapted my treatments so they can be carried out in the workplace, and offer the following fully clothed therapies to all office workers:

- Indian head massage

- Reiki master treatments
- Neck and shoulder massage
- Back massage
- Deep tissue massage
- Hand, wrist and arm massage
- Muscle energy technique (MET).

This treatment consists of a form of assisted stretching and breathing to lengthen muscles that have become tight or overused. It is one of the most effective treatments that can be carried out in the workplace to instantly relieve pain arising from tension and stress within minutes. Some of the organizations I have worked for include DEFRA, Oxleas NHS Trust and Ealing center for Independent Living and London Borough of Greenwich Council.

MUSCLE ENERGY TECHNIQUE (MET)

In essence, muscle energy techniques are a form of assisted stretching. For example, to stretch the hamstring, the therapist might raise the leg of the patient and place the ankle on his shoulder—The patient is then asked to press down on the shoulder, causing the hamstring to contract isometrically (Fig. V.6). Following on from this, the therapist should then be able to raise the leg beyond its previous limit—The exercise (also known as PNF stretching) can be repeated as necessary. Muscle energy techniques are very low risk, and can be used where high velocity thrusts are contraindicated.

Techniques

The massage techniques you will learn during this workshop include effleurage, petrissage, tapotement, hacking and cupping:

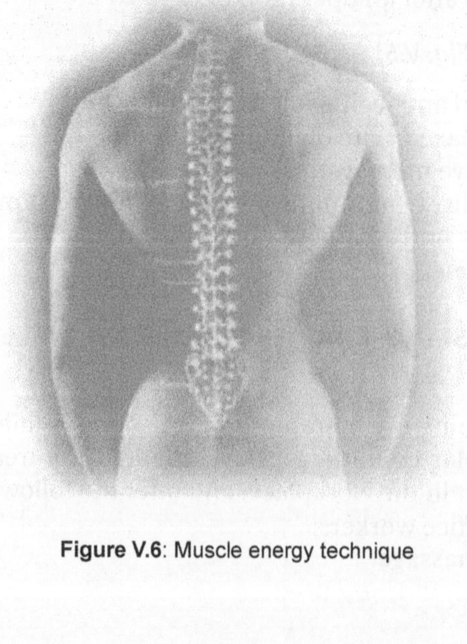

Figure V.6: Muscle energy technique

1. Effleurage: Gliding strokes with the palms, thumbs and/or fingertips
2. Petrissage: Kneading movements with the hands, thumbs and/or fingers
3. Tapotement: Gentle tapping over the face
4. Hacking: Using the side of the hands as a chopping movement
5. Cupping: Creating a cup-shape with your hands.

Techniques will be practised on each other so everyone gives and receives. The theory behind these techniques will be given during the workshop and general history of massage will be provided in the notes.

SPORT MASSAGE

Vigorous definitive strokes which loosen and warm up the muscles before and after exercise and help reduce lactic acid build-up on legs, back, shoulders and neck (Fig. V.7).

INDIAN HEAD MASSAGE

Indian head massage is an ancient form of massage originating from India and used in households from a very young age.

Indian head massage has now become popular in the West for its therapeutic uses, helping to relieve stress and tension from the shoulders, neck and head. Because it is concentrated on these areas it has a deeply relaxing effect on any muscular tension that often results in headaches, eyestrain and discomfort in the neck and shoulders (Fig. V.8).

Indian head massage not only works on a physical, but on an emotional level too, calming and refreshing the mind, promoting relaxation and peace. People often comment on feeling more focussed and uplifted after treatment as well as balanced and calm.

The treatment can be carried out fully clothed with no oils involved.

WHO AM I?

I am an ITEC qualified therapist and Reiki Master offering well-being

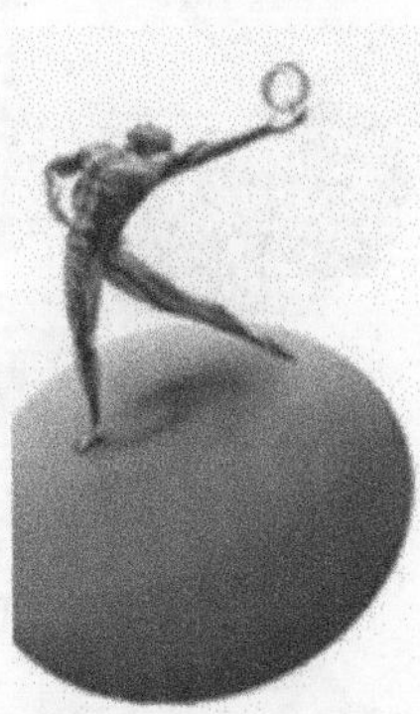

Figure V.7: Sport massage

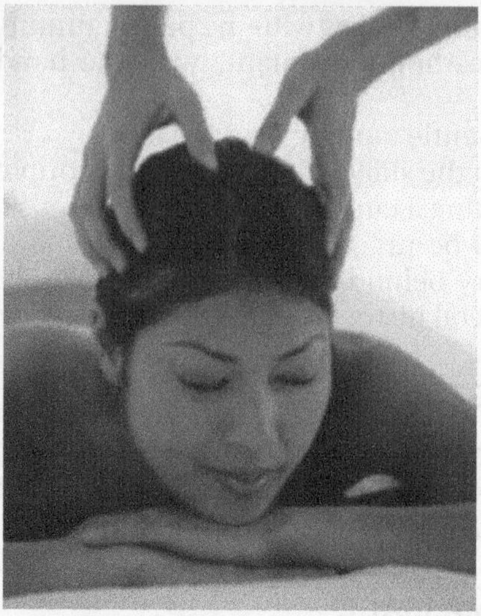

Figure V.8: Indian head massage

in the workplace. I have been treating clients with different muscle condition for over 8 years, and experienced in providing a combination of therapies to help them. I specialize in muscle energy technique (MET), and this technique is one of my most popular treatments for office workers (Fig. V.9).

WELL-BEING AT WORK

Recent findings from the Chartered Institute of Personnel and Development show that apart from minor illnesses such as colds and flus, the most common reason for employee absence were stress and

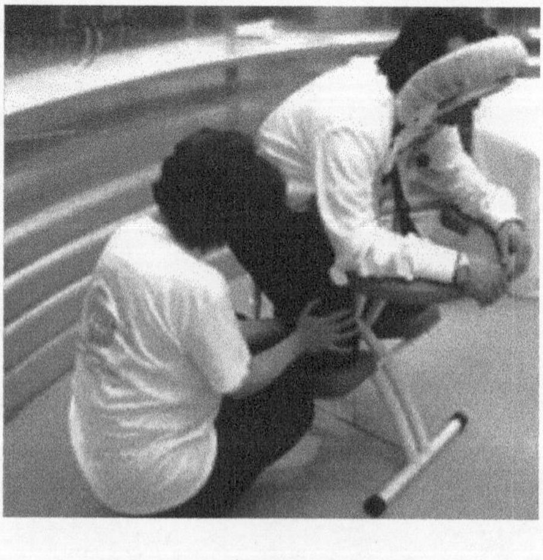

Figure V.9: Well-being at work

musculoskeletal disorders such as back and shoulder pain. Over 40% of the surveyed organizations said that stress-related illnesses had increased over the last year (Fig. V.9).

CONTRAINDICATIONS

There are times when massage could be detrimental rather than beneficial to you.

The contraindications to massage are:

- A body temperature over 100°F, or feeling unwell.
- Acute traumas— Open wounds, recent bruising, muscle tears, sprained ligaments, contusions, chilblains, burns.
- Tumors— Where there is swelling, which is inconsistent with recent bruising.
- Diseased blood vessels— Varicose veins, phlebitis, thrombosis
- Cancer
- Melanoma
- Hemophilia
- Infectious skin disease— Bacterial infection, lymphangitis, fungal infection, viral infections, herpes.
- Diabetes— Not strictly a contraindication, but massage has the same effect as exercise on your blood sugar levels so you need to have appropriate medication available.

If you have a medical condition it is advisable to seek advice from your consultant or doctor as many therapist will require a letter from your consultant or doctor if you have certain medical conditions.

UNIT-VI
Counseling

INTRODUCTION

It is a form of supportive psychotherapy in which the nurse and other qualified professional, such as licensed mental health counselors, offer guidance or assist the client in viewing option to problems that are discussed by the client in the context of the nurse-client relationship (ANA, 2000). The psychiatric mental health nurse must understand these dynamics while using counseling interventions or providing care to clients involved in psychotherapy.

According to the American Nurses Association (ANA, 2000) psychotherapy may be performed by the certified specialist in psychiatric mental health nursing. Psychotherapy may also be performed by licensed clinical social workers, clinical psychologists, and psychiatrists.

According to Shahrukh and Hales, 'Psychotherapy is a process in which a person who wishes to relieve symptoms, resolve problem in living, or seek personal growth enters into a contract to interact in a prescribed way with the psychotherapist.'

The psychiatric nurse uses counseling intervention to assist client in improving or regaining their previous coping abilities, fostering mental health, and preventing mental health, and mental illness and disability. Counseling interventions may occur in a variety of settings and may include the following:

- Communication and interviewing techniques
- Problem solving skills
- Stress management
- Crisis intervention
- Relaxation techniques
- Assertiveness training
- Conflict resolution
- Behavior modification.

Counseling is an important intervention during one-to-one interaction with clients or during the presentation of psychoeducation groups, medication groups and discharge planning groups. Client and their family members and significant others are given an opportunity to verbalize any concerns they may have. The counselors provide reassurance and clarification as the need arises.

Reassurance helps the client regain self-confidence and decreases feelings of guilt, anxiety and fear.

Clarification helps the client gain a clearer picture of reality by understanding feelings and behavior.

Explaining to a client with depression that the symptoms he or she in experiencing are related to a chemical imbalance in the brain that can be helped by antidepressants medication in an example of clarification of reality.

Counseling is meant for

Mild to moderate—

- Depression
- Relationship difficulties
- Anxiety
- Bereavement
- Emotional and psychological difficulties
- Response to physical illness
- Life cycle developmental issues
- Problem of adjustment
- Response to trauma
- Sexual difficulties.

GERIATRIC CARE COUNSELING

Geriatric care counseling is an independent care professional geriatric care management service which was established in 1994 for the purpose of assisting older adult and their families or other concerned parties in realistically assessing need and creating personalized plans tailor to meet the unique needs of each individual.

Geriatric care counseling is able to simplify and streamline the process of defining the needs of each senior and identifying the resources to best meet those needs.

What Services does Geriatric Care Counseling Provide?

- Family consultation
- In home personal needs assessment
- Creation of individual care plan
- Coordination of high quality home care services
- Evaluation of appropriate housing alternatives
- Crises management
- Excellent referrals for all types of community resources
- Care management services (short-term and long-term)
- Support for local and long distance relatives in need of assistance.

COUNSELING SERVICES FOR OLDER ADULTS

Although older adults have many strengths that may be called upon in times of need, some problems and losses may required outside help. For some people, painful event in the past, dissatisfaction in the present, or worries about the future may mean that they cannot enjoy life or achieve their goals. Adult children or others who are concerned about an older adult can also benefit from counseling services.

People who could benefit from counseling may be—

- Feeling depressed
- Adjusting to illness
- Experiencing stress in their families or social situation
- Having marital problems
- Grieving
- Concerned about or providing care for older adults.

TYPES OF COUNSELING SERVICES

- Individual counseling provides the opportunity to share problems with someone skilled in listening and helping people deal with problems or losses.
- Social worker counselors can work with people to set achievable goals and suggest ways of attaining those goals.
- They will also make referrals to other helping services if appropriate.
- Group counseling facilitated by skilled social workers provides participants the opportunity to give and receive emotional support from their peers.
- Problem solving is promoted through the sharing of mutual experiences.

The professional staff

- The counselors at geriatrics center are trained and qualified geriatrics social workers.
- They can work closely with physician and psychiatrists to provide care which takes into consideration the variety of health problems of individual clients.

Cultural sensitivity: Awareness of cultural and ethnic delivery in crucial to effective counseling. Therefore, unique needs of minority individuals are recognized and will be thoroughly addressed.

Scheduling appointments: Older adults or other concerned persons may call for a telephone interview about their needs and discuss what kind of services might be appropriate.

Confidentiality:

- Geriatrics center staff recognizes the confidential nature of the counseling process and will keep all information private.
- For U-M health system patients, a brief note including diagnosis, time spent, and progress towards a determined goal will be placed in the medical record.

Geriatric counseling,INC (GCI):

- Geriatric counseling provides assessment and counseling services to seniors and their families; living in long-term cure and isoresidential environment.
- GCI is one of the largest and most experienced providers of mental health services to seniors in the nation.
- GCI mental health clinicians are experts in geriatrics mental health issues.
- They can assess, identify and treat the problems which can interfere with the happiness the senior deserves in the life stage.
- It is committed to providing the greatest 'quality of life' care is the highest possible ethical and moral standards.

GCI provides a critical service and referral process are:

- Residents who have a mental health diagnosis listed on their face sheet.
- Residents who have care plans for mental health and behavioral issues.
- Residents who have on psychoactive medications.

And also provide:

- Psychological assessment.
- Psychotherapy.
- Behavioral management.
- Psychological testing.
- Interdisciplinary team consultation.
- Staff education family consultation.
- Administrative consultation.
- The transitions program focuses on senior family issues. A senior family is one that has a member who is experiencing issues related to aging.
- GCI provides assessment and counseling both to the family and work through this time of difficult change. These services are delivered in both outpatient and assisted living settings.

Counseling is available for the senior and their family members who are:

1. Experiencing difficulties with activities of daily livings (ADL'S)
2. Transitioning from home
3. Adjusting to new environments
4. Resolving family issues
5. Coping with mood changes
6. Dealing with changes in health
7. Improving interpersonal relationships.

ROLE OF NURSE IN GERIATRIC COUNSELING

Specially trained nurses can help upgrade resident care, but their use takes careful thought and planning in today's dynamic health care environment, all health care providers must use their resources creatively to remain competitive.

ROLE AND RESPONSIBILITIES IN GERIATRIC NURSING

- Integrate advanced knowledge and experience in delivering safe, effective quality care to geriatric clients in primary care.
- Demonstrate competence in managing the health/illness status of geriatric clients in primary care.
- Monitor and ensure quality health care delivery system on behalf of geriatric clients in primary care.
- Incorporate and understanding of trends in aging in planning and providing primary health care for clients.
- Demonstrate leadership and competence in implementing the role of primary care nurse practitioners.
- Engage in counseling, communication, collaboration and teaching in a manner that reflects caring, advocacy, ethics and professional standards.
- Conceptualize one's individuals role as a primary care nurse practitioner and one's personal philosophy of primary care practice.

The six subroles of the psychiatric nurse during a therapeutic relationship are as follows:

1. Nurse-teacher— The nurse-teacher educates clients about specifics illness and medication prescribed to promote stabilization of their condition.
2. Mother-surrogate— The nurturing need to clients who are unable to carry out simple tasks are met but the subrole of the mother-surrogate.
3. Technical nurse— The nurse manager is responsible for creating a therapeutic environment in which client feel safe and accepted.
4. Socializing agent— Social skills, such as interacting with others in a group setting, are promoted by the nurse who acts as a socializing agent.
5. Counselors/nurse therapist— The counselor or nurse therapist uses therapeutic skills to help clients identify and deal with stressors or problems that have resulted in dysfunctional coping.

PHASES OF A THERAPEUTIC RELATIONSHIP OF A NURSE

Therapeutic task accomplished by the psychiatric mental health nurse the initiating phase include:

- Build-up trust and rapport by demonstrating acceptance.
- Establishing a therapeutic environment, ensuring safe and privacy.
- Establishing a mode of communication acceptable to both client and nurse.
- Initiating a therapeutic contract by establishing a time, place and duration for each meeting as well as the length of time the relationship will be in effect.
- Assessing the client needs, coping strategies, defense mechanism, strength and weakness.

During the working phase include:
- Exploring the client perception of reality and providing constructive feedback.
- Helping client develop positive coping behaviors.
- Identifying available support system.
- Promoting a positive self-concept by focusing on what the client can do or not to do.
- Encouraging verbalization of feelings.
- Promoting clients independence by teaching new skills.
- Developing a plan of action with realistic goals.
- Implementing the plan of action.
- Evaluating the result of the plan of action.

During the termination phase:
- Provide self-care and maintain his or her environment.
- Demonstrate independence and work independently with others.
- Cope positively when experiencing feeling such as anxiety, anger, emotional stability.
- Identify the progress of the client.

BIBLIOGRAPHY

1. Rebraca SL. Basic Concepts of Psychiatric Mental Health Nursing, 7th ed, Lippincott: South Asian edition.
2. Ann BM. Psychiatric Nursing Contemporary practice, 4th ed. New Delhi, Lippincott: Wolters Kluwer (India) Pvt. Ltd.
3. Counseling service for older adults www.med.umich.edu/geriatrics
4. Geriatric counseling.INC.
5. mygic.com.

UNIT-VII
Psychiatric Rehabilitation

INTRODUCTION

Rehabilitation is the process of enabling the individual to return to his highest possible level of functioning. It is an important component of the community mental health program, and is taken at the level of tertiary prevention.

The utilization of the existing capacities of the handicapped person by the combined and coordinate use of medical, social, educational, and vocational measures to the optimum level of his functioning ability.

It is the process of minimizing the psychiatric impairment, the disabled person is helped to use his or her talents and to acquire confidence and self-esteem through experiencing success in social roles.

DEFINITION

According to Maxwell Jones, (1992) 'Rehabilitation is an attempt to provide the best possible community role which will enable the patient to achieve the maximum range of activity, interest and of which he is capable.'

AIMS

- Prevent chronic disabilities.
- Acquire and maintain the life skills that are necessary to cope up effectively.
- Helping the physically challenged and mentally challenged person to attain their best level of social functioning.
- The client will lead fully dependent life.
- Provide life-long support.

- Alleviates manifestations of problems is secondary.
- Improves client ego strength and ready to do any work independently.
- Cope up with emotional and interpersonal factors are involved in starting and continuation of work or job.

PRINCIPLES OF PSYCHIATRIC REHABILITATION

- It is a part of tertiary prevention; it is the limitation of disability related to an episode of an illness.
- It is a philosophy, an attitude—A state of mind, a mode of approach to treat the mental illness.
- Good rehabilitation requires skilled assessment of each client's potentialities.
- Reconstruction of the client's ego strengths, so that he can be made mentally fit and ready to work.
- To improve the capabilities and responsibilities, competencies of the person with psychiatric problems even the most disabled.
- It focuses on ability to function rather than developing a good insight.
- Utilizes a variety of therapeutic constructs.
- Improvement of vocational outcome.
- Emphasized on positive expectations, hope is the essential feature.
- An increase in independency levels.
- Active participation and involvement of clients in rehabilitation activities.
- Skill development, environmental resources development and functional interventions are the components of rehabilitation process.
- Comprehensive network of services recognizes and emphasize on continuity of care.
- Maximum use must be made of residual capacities.

REHABILITATION TEAM

- Psychiatrist
- Clinical psychologist
- Medicosocial worker
- Psychiatric nurse
- Counselor
- Occupational therapist
- Recreational therapist
- Other mental health care professionals.

APPROACHES OF PSYCHIATRIC REHABILITATION

Psychoeducation

After identification of underlying problems of mental illness, the team member will educate the client and his family members about the prognoses of illness, treatment alternatives; tries to clear unspoken fears, myths and prejudices by providing basic information and the care of the client in a context of respect and hope.

Include diagnosing the problem, telling the person what to expect regarding illness and discussing treatment alternatives.

Working with Families

The team members will utilize the family resources toward the welfare of the client. Families and other supporting agencies will be treated as partners in treatment and rehabilitation programs related to care and cure aspects. They will be involved actively in provision of care to the client.

Encouraging family members to get involved in treatment and rehabilitation programs.

Group Therapy

In psychiatric therapeutic modalities, group therapy is more effective than individual therapy as it provide opportunity to the client to develop social interaction, establishes interpersonal relationships by sharing their views, opinions related to problem solving abilities and techniques. The client will feel comfort in discussing about their problems and its solution.

Positive aspect of group therapy includes an opportunity for ongoing contacts with others, validation of their perceptions, sharing their views about problem and problem solving abilities.

Social Skills

The team member will teach the client about the living skills, communication skills and other social skills which are required to the client to live happily within the community settings. It includes the abilities required for normal social interaction, expression of emotional feelings, employment and vocational skills, management of money, household activities and other modalities related to hygiene, therapeutic modalities, follow-up and continuity of care-related to promotion of mental health and prevention of mental illness.

It involves teaching specific living skills that the patient is expected to have in order to survive in the community.

STEPS IN PSYCHIATRIC REHABILITATION

Psychiatric rehabilitation begins with a comprehensive medical psychiatric diagnosis and functional assessment. These are key elements in identifying impairments and disabilities. The steps of rehabilitation include:

1. **Reduction of impairment**: Rehabilitation interventions with psychiatric patients require reduction or elimination of the

symptoms and cognitive impairments that interfere with social and vocational performance. This impairment are reduced and eliminated for the greater part by various psychotropic agents.

2. **Remediation of disabilities through skill training**: Skill training is used to remediate disabilities in social, family and vocational functioning. Patients generally require training in self-care skills, interpersonal skills, vocational and employment pursuits, recreational and leisure skills.
3. **Remediating disabilities through support intervention**: When restoration of social and vocational functioning through skills training is limited by continuing deficits, rehabilitation strategies aim at helping the individual compensate for handicap by learning skills in living and working environments, adjusting the individual and family expectations to a level of functioning that is realistically attainable.
4. **Remediation of handicaps**: In addition to clinical rehabilitation interventions, the disabled persons can be helped to overcome their handicaps through social rehabilitation interventions, for example, community support programs.

TYPES OF REHABILITATION

Social Rehabilitation

To reinculcate interaction and establish effective social relationship to overcome social barriers and to return to the normative life within the community, social rehabilitation is required. The client has to feel a sense of responsibility and adapt healthy roles and modifies the deviant behavior with normal behavior. The preventive and curative measures will be adopted by the individual client to lead satisfactory and unusual life in social environment. Opportunities have to be provided to the client to maintain and reestablish social adequacy in the life.

Educational Rehabilitation

Educating or giving training for as person with a psychiatric disorder in specific areas is essential whereby the client meets the goals of treatment and rehabilitation. For example, explaining the client and his family about client's disease condition and its prognosis, treatment alternatives: fears and myths associated with it: giving proper explanation and reality goals. Remedial education related to vocational service in supportive environment is provided. Encourage the clients who have the capabilities to undergo higher education and attainment of vocational skills. Measures are taken to enhance the person's acceptance of his illness; encourage the client and family members to actively participate in care-related activities and adopt coping strategies to overcome the problems occurring related to disease process and to live more productively within the community.

Occupational Rehabilitation

It will be carried out to achieve job-oriented skills and pleasure seeking activities, whereby the client obtain independent way of living and will try to overcome the problems related to illness.

Vocational Rehabilitation

Vocational rehabilitation is a part of continuous and coordinate process of rehabilitation which involve the provision of those vocational services (e.g. vocational guidance, vocational training and selective placement) designed to enable a disabled person secure and retain suitable employment.

Specialized services like counseling, vocational guidance, vocational training, developing adequate work tolerance, work social skills and job findings, placement, follow-up services and continuity of care will be provided. Vocational rehabilitation team includes psychologist, psychiatrists, medicosocial workers, nurses and relatives. Each client has different levels of adjustment to his environment.

AIMS

- Modification of attitudes may avoid relapses
- Promotion of mental health
- Timely help, acceptance, positive and sympathetic attitude, etc. arrests further deterioration
- Family members will be involved in decision making and active participation in provision of care
- Provides emotional support and task oriented assistance
- Aids access to social contact
- Fully utilize the inherent potentials.

INDICATIONS

- Persons who lost their jobs due to disease process
- Early onset of illness and lack/deprived of education and training opportunities
- Clients who were left with residual psychiatric problems.

PRINCIPLES

The international labor organization in 1979 formulated the principles for mentally restored persons. Mentally restored are, 'the client who were recovered from mental illness and is ready to receive vocational assistance (vocational preparation, training, evaluation and employment)'.

- The disabilities, social circumstances have to be considered.
- As rehabilitation is a form of social learning, educational element plays a vital role.

- Maintain social contact with the network of social relationships.
- Involve the hospital staff and labor services, local employment offices in finding out the vocational resource.
- Integrate the services for both physically disabled and mentally restored.
- Medical treatments are integrated with a structured program of various resources.
- Creates legal framework to ensure job security for the mentally challenged individual to facilitate vocation resettlement.

The vocational rehabilitation program includes the following components:

- Open competitive job placement
- Sheltered employment
- Self-employment
- Home-bound work programs
- Follow-up continuity of services.

COMPONENTS OF VOCATIONAL REHABILITATION

Open Competitive Job Placement

Indications

- Reactive psychosis
- Manic depressive psychosis with infrequent attacks.
- Acute psychotic episodes
- With regular follow-up programs, guidance and counseling services can function effectively and able to perform their abilities and duties successfully.

Sheltered Employment

Indications

- Mental retardation
- Chronic illness, e.g. schizophrenia, repeated attacks of affective disorders, irregular medication usage.

These cases cannot cope with ordinary employment. They will be given an opportunity to work under supervision, i.e. in rehabilitation homes.

Self-employment

Indications

- Mentally restored persons
- Mentally retarded

- Residual schizophrenia
- MDP.

Social welfare departments, small scale industrialists will have the facility/provision of sanctioning of loans for self-employment scheme; if the mentally restored persons are unable to cope-up with the demand of vocational adjustment in the open competitive job situations, but who have the capacity to do some work, in those cases family members will come forward and provide necessary support for self-employment of the client; with that moral support work output, income improvement, feelings of acceptance and security, etc. will be strengthened for mentally restored clients.

Home-bound Work Programs

Indications

Chronically mentally ill cases—These type of programs were based on the setting of urban or rural and the rehabilitation potentials availability within the family and community for acquiring the feelings of acceptance. Rural areas will provide better rehabilitation scope than the urban areas, where high skill and preparation is needed for job.

Depending upon the capacities, abilities of mentally restored persons the work activities will be allotted to the client like gardening, crafts, cattle rearing, sheep breeding, agriculture activities, etc. will be provide in the rural areas. For chronic cases they will be asked to help in the household activities, keeping cattle shed clean, carrying food for the people in job, whatever he is capable to do, that type of work will be allotted.

Follow-up Program and Continuity of Care

It is a linking program between intensive treatment and a complete session of treatment.

Indications

- When an inpatient and outpatient program is completed.
- In some cases relapses are common, hence follow-up care is essential.

Aims

- Follow-up program will help the client to gradually withdraw from the treatment process.
- To get himself to the family environment after hospitalization.

TIPS TO PROMOTE FOLLOW-UP SERVICES

- Therapeutic relationship has to be established between the client, family members and therapeutic team members.

- Orientation training program and to enhance their knowledge (client and family members about disease process, manifestations, treatment and possible side effects of the drugs) follow-up of the client.
- Involve the family members to supervise the client's activities, after administration of the medications for any side effects of drug intake.
- To enhance treatment adherence, provide family counseling and situational support, and implementing therapeutic activities and by sharing responsibility in regular follow-up care activities.
- Gather details from the family members, if any untoward effect observed during implementation of therapeutic activities; instruct the family members to seek advice from the nearby health care institutions.
- Regular home visit by community psychiatric nurse or reminding letters or through interaction with other client's who have improved from their illness will motivate the client to go for regular checkups or follow-up services for improving their conditions.
- Involve personal involuntary organizations, formal and informal leaders and teachers for motivating client's family for treatment adherence of the client.
- Frequency of appointment for the client to the clinic, transport facilities and traveling concessions for the client and family members accompanying will enhance the follow-up visits.
- Accessibility of health centers, availability of health centers, availability of health professional, immediate implementation of interventions will enhance follow-up services.

RE-EMPLOYMENT OPPORTUNITIES

In the urban community either government agencies or private sectors will assist in providing re-employment for the employees from sheltered workshop. For small scale industries, agencies will ensure supply for all essential and scarce raw materials. Finance facilities for banks, concession towards interests. 100% income tax exemption, job reservation quota, family pension, subsidized facilities, etc. are provided.

PHASES IN VOCATIONAL REHABILITATION

- Vocational assessment
- Vocational counseling
- Vocational training
- Job exploration
- Job placement
- Follow-up.

Vocational Assessment

It is done in four areas, i.e. clinical, social, psychological and vocational.

- Clinical assessment includes assessing for residual psychiatric symptoms which may affect his ability to function.
- Support assessment includes assessing family support, attitude of family members and economic status of the family.
- Psychological assessment includes assessing self-esteem, confidence, and patient's level of motivation.
- Vocational assessment includes assessing physical strength, hand co-ordination, attention, concentration, etc.

Vocational Counseling

This includes informing patients and family members regarding the type of training available. Family consent should be taken for rehabilitation training.

Vocational Training

It includes:
- Course content
- Duration of training
- Incentives
- Assessment of the progress
- Imparting skills
- Supervision.

Job Exploration

Finding out various jobs available in the community.

Job Placement

This includes selecting suitable job, placement of the patient in the job, checking the facilities available and evaluating work performance.

Follow-up

It includes evaluation of the four dimensions, i.e. clinical, social, psychological, and vocational.

VOCATIONAL PROGRAM

Open competitive job placement: Though it is difficult to place the mentally restored in open competitive job placements, it is also possible to provide this opportunity for selected group of patients with clinical diagnosis of reactive psychosis, bipolar affective disorders, and acute psychotic episodes. They can be equipped to function successfully by regular follow-up programs.

Sheltered employment: This is provided for those disabled persons, who because of the nature and severity of the disability, cannot cope with ordinary employment. This is suitable for those with the problem of mental retardation, chronic mental illness (e.g. schizophrenia, repeated attacks of affective disorder in spite of regular medication).

Self-employment: Person who cannot cope with the demand of vocational adjustment in open competitive job situations, but who have the capacity to do some work with the help of any family members, may be considered for self-employment schemes which are usually sponsored by different welfare schemes of nationalized banks and social welfare departments.

Home-bound work programs: For those disabled need total care, work can be given at home, which shall be collected by the center and paid according to the performance.

DIFFICULTIES IN REHABILITATION

- To find wholesome environment, adequate housing for the client to live comfortably.
- To identify job resources and to find out suitable job.
- Unable to participate actively, occupationally and socially in the life.
- The attitude of family members will be affecting the client's performance related to instrumental and expressive functions of the family.

ROLE OF NURSE IN REHABILITATION

Rehabilitation psychiatric nursing must be studied in the context of both the patient and social system. This requires focusing on three elements, the individual, the family and community.

Rehabilitation psychiatric nursing focuses in context with individual (client) and social system (family and community). The care is related to activities of nursing process, i.e. assessment, planning, implementation, evaluation.

Assessment

Assessment of the individual

It begins with the initial contact between the patient and the nurse. It helps to understand the client's potentialities/strengths; limitation in detail and nurse can help them to achieve maximum possible functioning at the earliest with proper planning and implementation of the nursing interventions to the client in order to promote healthy lifestyle. Nurses identify the stressers that may interfere with the client's adjustment process and provide appropriate support by utilizing coping strategies and adapt suitable treatment techniques. Nurse has to assess the individual in the following areas:

- The activities of the daily living: To live independently; and for successful functioning of the individual within the community. The main aim of the rehabilitation is to assist the person to develop independent living skills. The ADL includes housekeeping, shopping and food preparation, personal hygiene and money management, learning working skills. Nurse identifies the strengths, establish goals and set priorities for skill development.

- Interpersonal relationship: How the person is able to develop good IPR with the family members and other fellow beings are observed.
- Self-esteem: The feeling of self-worth and regards to one self.
- Motivation abilities, Strength/abilities/skills/interests related to leisure activities, recreational skills, work skills, educational accomplishments, special interests, talents, etc. have to be observed.
- Adherence pattern: For example following instructions and utilizing coping strategies will improve the condition, aids in progress in rehabilitation process.
- Nonadherence pattern: Not following the instructions. For example if treatment modalities are not followed sometime rehospitalization occur.
- Drug compliance: Acceptance for drug and able to observe drug actions, side effects and take proper precautions while consuming drugs or not.

Assessment of the family

Family resources are assessed, before rehabilitation plan is developed as family members have a right to provide input in the treatment plan and they are the best person to identify the problematic areas and enhance in implementing measures to the client's compliance to the plan.

Components

- Family structure: Type of family and size and developmental roles and responsibilities, norms, values.
- Family attitude toward the mentally sick.
- Emotional climate of the family, e.g. fearful, calm, depress, etc.
- Social support to the family, e.g. friends, relatives, financial support, religious and community support.
- Past family experiences with mental health services.
- Family understanding of client's problems and plan of care.

Assessment of the community

Identification of community agencies which will come forward to provide services to people with mental illness. Collaborative relationships between health care providers and community agencies are essential part of rehabilitation.

Planning and Implementation

To maximize personal strengths and foster independence. Nurse, client and his family work together to overcome any remaining impaired areas of functioning.

Individual interventions

Remove impairment and disabilities and to improve social and vocational performance and cognitive abilities of an individual, rehabilitation intervention are carried out with the people of psychotropic agents and case management.

Skill training

It will be used to remediate the disabilities in social, family and vocational functioning. In the following areas, skill training are given like self-care skills, leisure skills, interpersonal skills and vocational skills.

Supportive interventions

Learning and living and working skills which are required in living situation will help the individual to lead a satisfied family life according to their expectations and realistic way of living.

Community supportive programs

As a part of social rehabilitation activity, community support programs and arranged.

Vocational rehabilitation activities

To develop independent skills and to maximize individual strengths, vocational guidance, training, selective placement (open competitive jobs, sheltered employments, home-bound work programs) are provided. Disabled persons are secured with suitable employment.

Family interventions

- Family therapy
- Group therapy
- Family counseling
- Supportive psycho-educational therapy
- Health team campaigns about disease process, available resources and problem solving techniques
- Self-help groups
- Community-based rehabilitation services or support programs are carried out
- Crises intervention programs
- Outreach programs.

Community interventions

Providing care of the client in community settings, e.g. halfway homes, residential prevention programs are carried out within the community.

Utilize the community activities like volunteers school teachers, paraprofessional in taking care of mentally sick (Fig. VII.1).

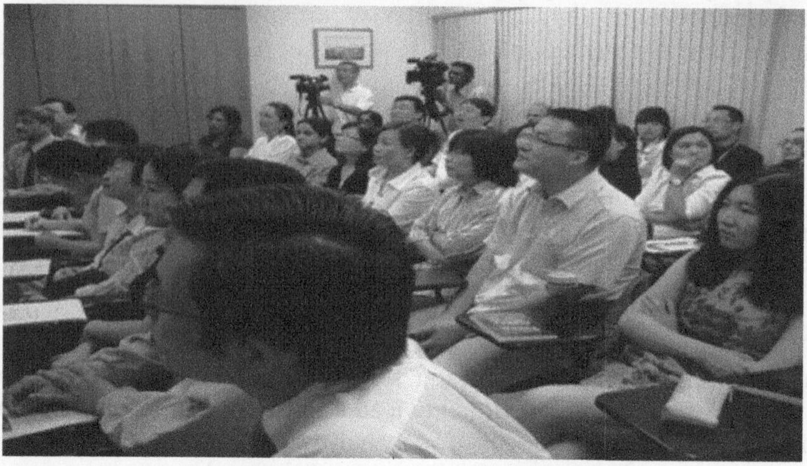

Figure VII.1: Community intervention

Evaluation

The client's adjustment, family adaptation and effectiveness of the community service system are evaluated in psychiatric rehabilitation services.

REHABILITATION SERVICES IN INDIA

One of the important recommendation of World Health Organization (WHO, 2001) has been to develop community-based mental health care program. In India, the national human rights commission pointed out the need of management of growing chronic population and stress the demand for providing rehabilitation activity in all hospital the Supreme Court has also directed to involve NGOs the process of rehabilitation in the hospitals. In India for a population of approximately 1 billion people, the psychiatric disorder like schizophrenia is prevalent in an estimated 4 million peoples an estimated 60% of them require rehabilitation on their road to recovery (WHO, 2001). Taking thumb rule of ten, it has been estimated that about 20% to 25% of those ill with severe mental disorders need long-term rehabilitation. Thus today a large proportion of person with mental illness and mood disorder experience a poor quality of life with long-term disability, persisting symptoms, or a relapsing course of illness which has given birth to the field of psychiatric and psychological rehabilitations in India.

Rehabilitation services in mental health are delivered through hospital meetings and community involvement.

Rehabilitation Facilities at Hospitals

The major findings for psychiatric rehabilitation activities revealed that only 36% of government mental hospitals have a separate facility for vocational training. The rehabilitation activities were confined to the occupational unit.

Rehabilitation facilities at community

The birth of psychological rehabilitation gave momentum for the community-based rehabilitation program. Some of the NGOs run rehabilitation centers are—

- Half way homes
- Home medicopastoral association
- CADBAM Bangalore
- Family day care center
- Long stay homes
- Jyoti niwas
- Biopsychosocio model, Pune
- Day care services, Sarthaj
- Sheltered workshop, Ashadeep.
- Self-help group like Margdarshika
- ASHA at Chennai
- Richmond fellowship in Banglore
- SCARF, Chennai
- SHRISTI, Madurai
- PRERNA, Mumbai
- SAMARPAN, Indore
- BPA, Ahmedabad
- ASHAADEEP, Janagadha
- VARDAAN day care center
- Others centers.

Model of psychiatric rehabilitation center

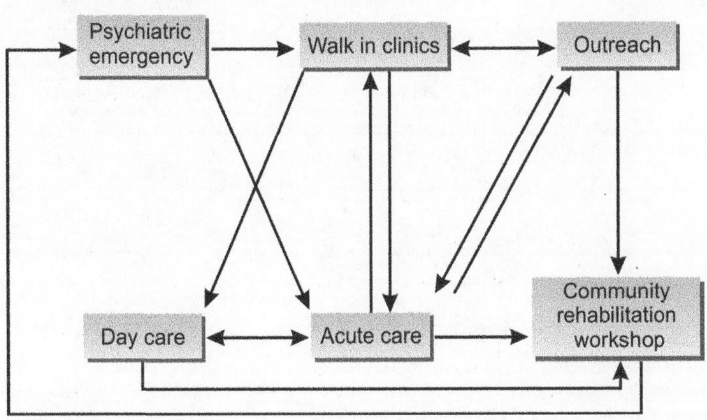

MAIN VOCATIONAL REHABILITATION CENTERS IN INDIA

- Mithra Special School and Vocational Center for mentally retarded, Chennai.
- Banyan, Chennai.
- Vocational Rehabilitation Center, Chennai.
- Shristi Center for Psychiatric Rehabilitation, Madurai.
- VTC (vocational training center) for the physically handicapped, run by the Ministry of Labor, Government of India, has opened up its facility for the mentally ill for the first time in Chennai.
- Indian Red Cross Society which runs VTC for the handicapped has offered vocational training for the chronically ill.
- Indian Council for Child Welfare, and NGOs caring for underprivileged children.

Index

T